Native American Indigenous Church INC

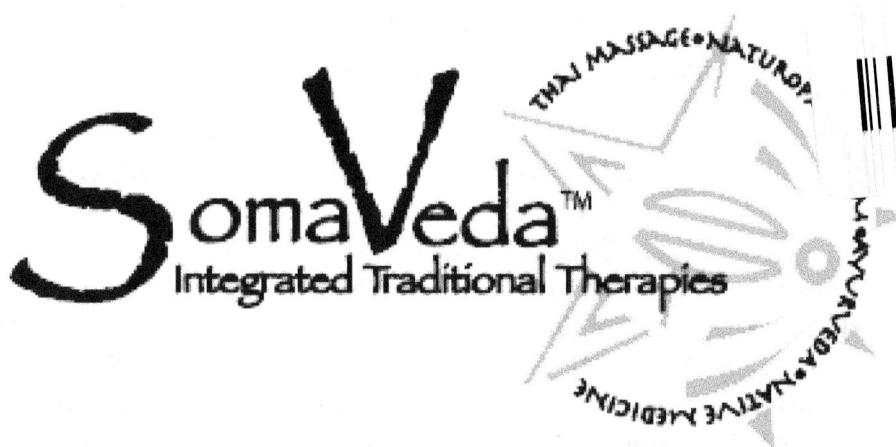

SomaVeda™
Integrated Traditional Therapies

Ayurvedic Thai Yoga:

Indigenous Religious Therapeutics and Traditional Medicine

Anthony B. James

SomaVeda® Level Two...The Southern Method

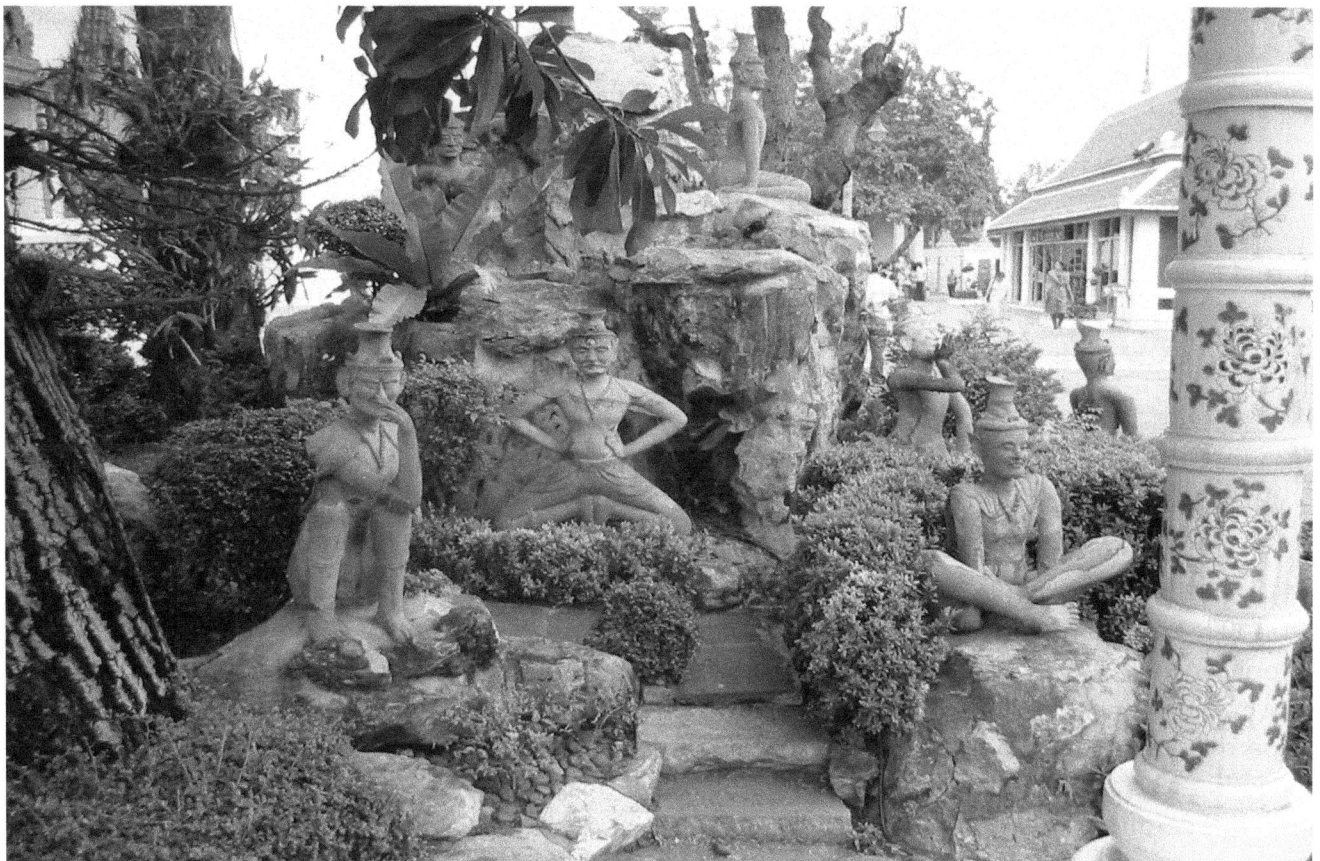

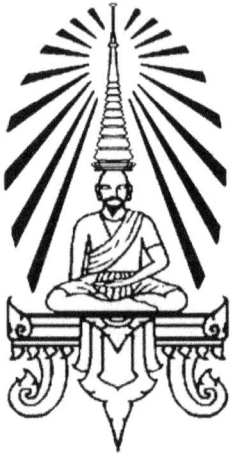

Native American Indigenous Church

Ayurvedic Thai Yoga

Indigenous Religious Therapeutics and Traditional Medicine

SomaVeda® Level Two Workbook

Anthony B. James

5401 Saving Grace Ln. Brooksville, FL 34602

(706)358-8646,

e-mail nativeaic@somaveda.com

Web Site: ThaiYogaCenter.Com

SomaVeda.Com

SomaVeda.Org

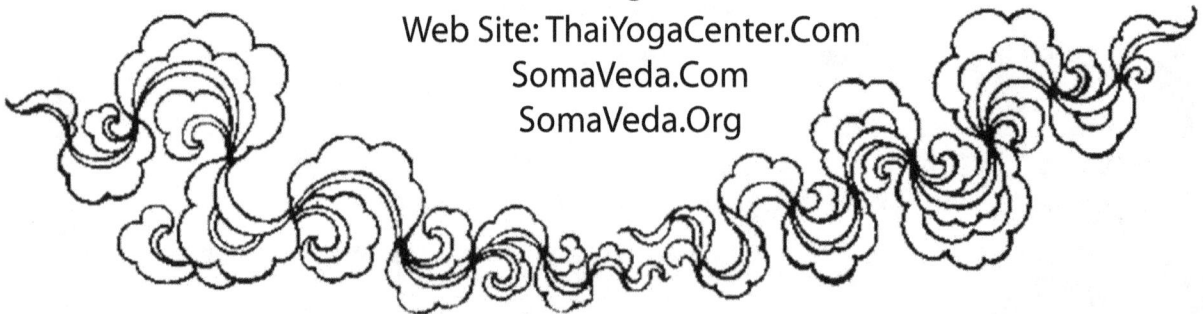

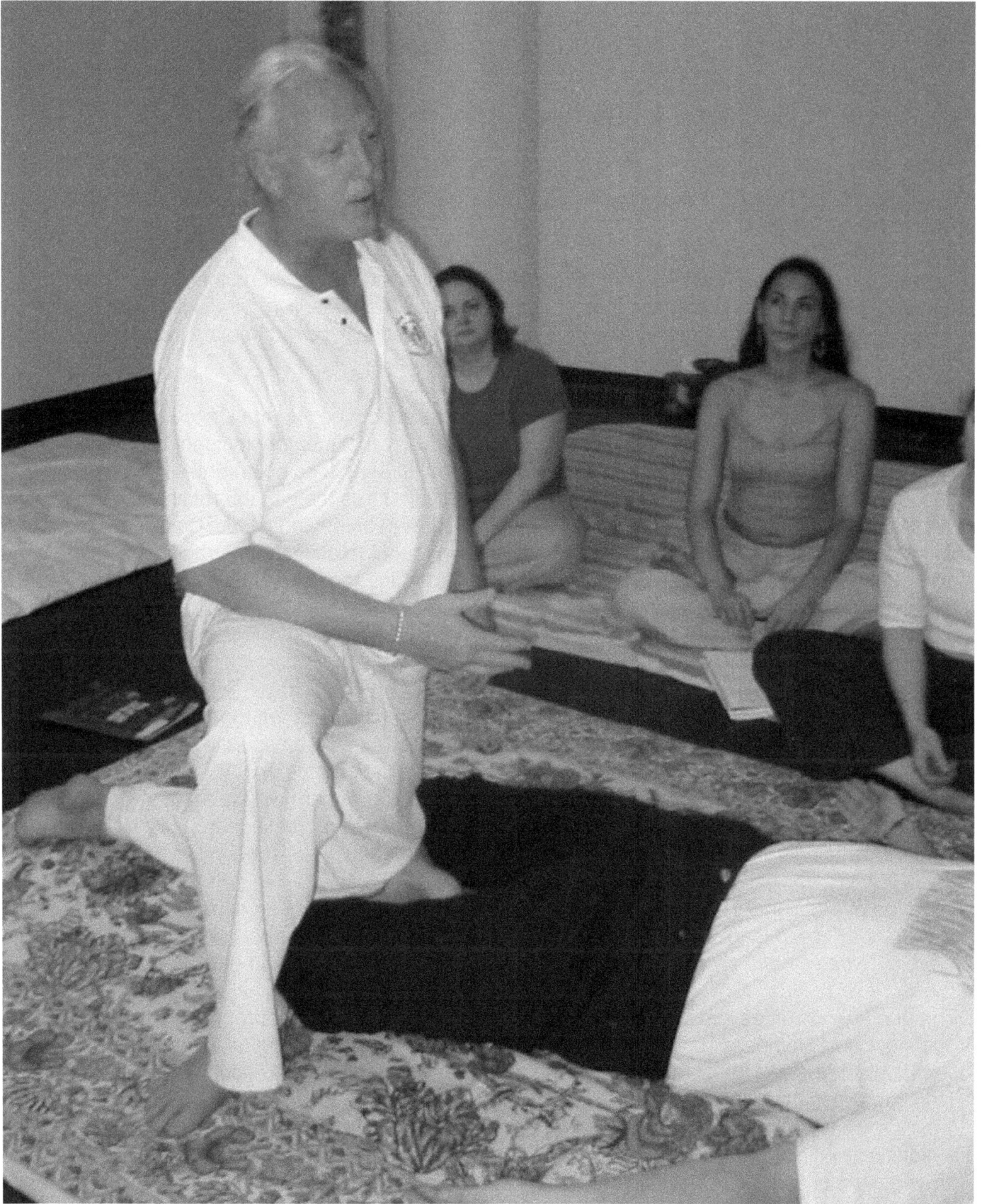

Ajahn James presents "Fa Meung" , Palm Pressing technique for the medial upper leg. (NY 2004)

Please Note: This material is the companion and supplemental workbook to the primary SomaVeda® Level Two textbook "Ayurveda of Thailand: Indigenous Traditional Thai Medicine and Yoga Therapy" by Anthony B. James, Meta Journal Press, Brooksville, FL 34602 (Available on BeardedMedia.com and Amazon.Com)

What Is Indigenous Traditional Thai Yoga or "Thai Massage- slang"?

Thai Yoga is comprehensive, sophisticated healing arts derivative of Theraveda Buddhism, Buddhist medicine, Buddhist Psychology, Theraveda Vipassana Bhavana, Classical Indian and Tibetan Ayurveda, and Yoga Vedanta.

Indigenous Traditional Thai Yoga (I.T.T.M.) is an ancient system of religious therapeutics based on Ayurveda, Buddhist medicine, and indigenous, traditional Tribal Medicine practices. It has been developed and practiced as a sacred, spiritual, and energetically based healing system for thousands of years, first in India and then in Thailand to the present day.

PLEASE NOTE: In 1983, Ajahn, Dr. Anthony B. James introduced it to the United States. Today it is practiced widely and has been formally incorporated as a complimentary indigenous medicine system by the Native American Indigenous Church, Inc. (NAIC). It complements all Native American and indigenous traditional medicine and healing practices. It fills the gap in practical ministry, sacred medicine, and healing knowledge lost to Native American peoples and culture due to past excesses, diaspora, and genocide. Since 1992 I.T.T.M. has been taught to indigenous, traditional Native medicine men and women as a practical expression of Indigenous and Native American Religion and Religious Therapeutics (Aboriginal Medicine). In the US, the religious expression and traditional medicine practices of Native Americans and Indigenous persons are protected by US Federal Code (AIRFA/RLUIPA) and International Treaty (UNDRIP).

Becoming a Hindu or Buddhist is not required to practice this healing art, though it is helpful to understand Ayurveda and or Buddhist medicinal principles. It is more accurate to call this medicine by its traditional names like "ancient, anachronistic, or Old Indigenous Thai Way of Healing with The Hands." However, the slang form "Thai Massage" is in use, and there will be some understandable confusion as long as this is so. We recommend that ministers and practitioners, as medicine persons, refrain from or NOT use the term "Thai Massage" to avoid misunderstanding and confusion.

The type of traditional Thai Yoga therapy that most people will have been exposed to is *"ráksãa thaang nûat"* (healing massage treatment). *"ráksãa thaang nûat"* is commonly known as the *"Nuat Thai"* or *"Nuad Boran"* styles of Thai Yoga therapy, spiritual massage, and healing work of Thailand.

The primary outcomes associated with Thai Yoga are ProMiiWihan Sii or four divine, boundless states of mind; Love, Compassion, Joy, and Equanimity. It is successful as long as these four qualities are communicated, transmitted, and exemplified during a session. For this reason, it is possible to have a Thai Yoga session with little or no actual touching!

In addition to the four divine states of mind, we practice and perform "*Puja*"- a ritual healing process of prayer, affirmation, and acknowledgment. We acknowledge the sacred space shared by the client and therapist, we honor and acknowledge the Bodhisattvas and progenitors of our way and teaching, and we "generate the Boddichitta," the perfected mental processes of enlightened beings through Mantra recitation of "*OmNamoShivago*", the Metta Sutra, or anything else that invokes and invites the essence and energy of love and healing to move within ourselves and our client.

This prayerful and thoughtful meditation attunes powerful energies and petitions the sacred and symbolic metaphors of deities, ancient guides, and role models that provide the basis for all further communication and expression of *"ProMiiWihan Sii."*

The secondary outcomes are of lesser importance and may or may not share characteristics common to many forms of Western massages, such as effleurage (stroking and kneading the muscles), manipulation (manipulating or aligning osseous or skeletal parts) and pressure point or acupressure style technique (applying deep, consistent pressure to specific nerves, tendons, or ligaments, acupoints, *"Marma"* or *"Thai Lom"*).

In order to balance the functions of the four body elements called *"thâat tháng sìi"* (*Lom, Fai, Din, Naam*), Thai Yoga incorporates elements of prayer (sacred affirmations), energetic, Prana, Dosha assessment, mindfulness, gentle rocking, Asana positional release, deep stretching, focused breathing or Prana Yama, Chakra balancing, Prana Nadi or Sen line balancing and rhythmic compression to create a singular healing experience.

The Native American Indigenous Church, Inc. (N.A.I.C.) and the Thai Yoga Center represent and support authentic Indigenous Traditional Thai Medicine (I.T.T.M.), Thai culture, and healing arts. Even though we are founded as a Native American Church, we recognize and validate the indigenous and natural medicine of native peoples, including Indigenous Thai People, as an expression of Mother Earths' gifts for healing and well-being.

Our instructors are directly authorized teachers, representatives, and traditional lineage holders in several different traditional secular and traditional Buddhist schools:

-Buddhai Sawan Institute Ayudthaya and Nongkam (famous for martial and healing arts for centuries)
-Phra Wat Chetuphon (Buddhist Temple, Wat Po Traditional Thai Medical School...One of the oldest
    schools of traditional arts),
- U.T.T.S. (Union of Thai Traditional Medicine Society, Royal Thai Ministry of Health)
-Buntautuk Hilltribes Northern Provincial Hospital and Training Institute, also known as "The Old
    Medicine Hospital of Shivago Komarpai."
-ITM (International Thai Massage, Chiangmai)
-Mama Lek Chaiya:Nerve Touch (Jap Sen Nuad) Lanna Tradition, Chiangmai
Lanna School of Thai Massage: Chiangmai
-The Foundation for the Blind -Buddhist Temple Wat Sawankholok, School for the Blind
-Wangklaikangwon Industrial Community & Educational College program sponsored by
    HM. King Bhumibol, Anantasuk School of Thai Traditional Medicine)

There are several other significant lineages, teachers, and Grand Masters. Most important is the Buddhist medicine derived from the famous Saint Shivago (Jivaka). In the United States, traditional lineage and teaching are passed on via the Thai Yoga Center educational programs for SomaVeda Integrated Traditional Therapies® in Brooksville, FL. Additionally, we recognize all schools formally recognized by the Royal Thai Ministries of Health and of Education and The Union of Thai Traditional Medicine Society (U.T.T.S.) listed or not!

Many traditional "schools" of Indigenous Traditional Thai yoga therapy (I.T.T.M.) exist. They range from the big university-driven or supported programs of Bangkok to the "family" style oral and traditional lineages of the Northern Hill Tribe people such as Karen, Lisu, Lahu, Mien, and Akha. Their influence is a growing factor in the modern expression of Thai Yoga, especially in the North.

Indigenous Traditional Thai Yoga (I.T.T.M.) is a colloquial or geographically distinctive system. Modern Thai yoga therapy synthesizes several different regional variations based on location, region, and in some cases, the specific influence of a charismatic teacher. Traditionally there was mention of the "Seven Schools." Of course, there were not in the past only seven schools! Considering this was the primary medicine of millions of people for over a thousand years, it is logical to assume there were many different schools in operation at one time or another. For example, every temple teaching or practicing these healing arts could have been considered a school, and there were hundreds, if not thousands of these over the years.

The most famous traditional school in the North is The Buntautuk Northern Hill Tribe Medical Hospital or "The Old Medicine Hospital." Under Grand Master Ajahn Sintorn Chaichagun (Transitioned November 2005), it has become a national and international phenomenon. Teaching various levels of programs to Thai and falang (foreigners) alike, Ajahn Sintorn was also famous for his daily recitation of the Pali Om Namo Shivago prayer and invocation for blessing. Twice daily, he would lead the entire community in this rhythmic and beautiful traditional mantra for healing. In the North, they say, "You do not know Thai Yoga Therapy until you know this mantra!" Today the Wat Po Association of Traditional Doctors, member schools, and Aachans or Master Instructors are bringing this work into the modern world. Famous schools and their head Masters, such as Anantasuk Rongrian under both Phaa Kruu Anantasuk and Ajahn Nantipa Anantasuk, work with the King's "*Rajaprajanugroh*" projects to thoroughly document the traditional medicine and preserve its rich heritage.

Northern Thailand is closer to mainland China so there are more Chinese and Laotion-influenced massage techniques. For example, a well-known teacher and practitioner in Chiangmai, Grand Master, Mama Lek Chaiya, and her family were famous for teaching the Wat Suandok style known as *"nûat jàp sên"* (nerve-touch massage), a Chinese-style acupressure technique that works with the body's nerve meridians, much like acupuncture. Some plucking techniques are reminiscent of Tuina and can be pretty unpleasant. However, the ultimate aim of balancing the chi takes precedence over comfort!

It is important to remember that all applications of physical pressure are intended to convey ProMiiwihan Sii to balance and harmonize the *"thâat tháng sìi"* and Tri_dosha or Three Winds, Humors or energetically based body types. Thai yoga is a sophisticated system of Ayurveda exchanging love with pressure, just as a hug can convey care, consideration, and love with physical pressure. In Thai Yoga (I.T.T.M.), a loving embrace is conveyed with great detail and sophistication.

The practice of Thai Yoga is substantially based on principles of classical Ayurveda as described in the classic Ayurveda Medicine texts: Caraka Samhita, Atchara Veda, Gheranda Samhita, Pradipika, and Ramayana, without most of the overt references to Hindu deities. Ayurvedic practices emphasized in Thai yoga include Samkhya (Sanskrit= Satkhya), Creation Cosmology, Rajas, Satvas and Tamas, Dhatus, Doshas, Sen Lines (Prana Nadi), Lom (Wind Gates, Sanskrit= Marma), Pancha Karma, Asana, Prana Yama, and Mantra. The philosophies and principles of these Ayurvedic texts have also been re-interpreted in Theraveda Buddhism. Two influential texts in the Theraveda system are the Buddha Dharma and the Vipassana Bhavana.

The four Thai Ayurvedic elements are **Earth** (din-solid parts of the body, including nerves, skeleton, muscles, blood vessels, tendons, and ligaments); **Water** (*náam*-blood and bodily secretions); **Fire** (*fai*-digestion and metabolism); and **Air** (Ether/Aether, "*lom*"-respiration, and circulation). Borrowing from India's Ayurvedic tradition, some practitioners employ Pali-Sanskrit terms for the four bodily elements: pathavidhatu, apodhatu, tecodhatu, and vayodhatu. The book "Lines, Wheels, Points and Specific Remedies" covers this theory in detail. Indigenous Traditional Thai Yoga Therapy and or "Traditional Thai massage" are systems of yoga therapy, and all aspects of Somaveda® Thai Yoga follow Ayurvedic and yogic principles.

From the very first origins of what was to become Thailand, from the Srisatchanali, Sukhotai, and Ayutthaya periods right to the present day, the Thai government's Departments and or Ministries of Health included an official massage division (phanâek mãw nûat). Under the influence of international Medicine and modern hospital development, the responsibility for the national propagation/ maintenance of temple-based Thai Ayurveda (Ayurveda of Thailand) was eventually transferred to Phra Wat Chetaphon (Wat Pho) in Bangkok, where it remains today. Traditional Yoga therapy has persisted in most provinces, and there has recently been a resurgence of popularity throughout the country. The Wat Po system is divided into two separate and distinctive categories: the tourist massage pavilion and Tourist massage school (*Rongrian Sala Thaang Nuaat*) and the School for traditional Medicine for training and certification of "*Maw Nuad phaen boran Thaï*" (Massage Doctors). There are considerable differences in the term and quality of training. For example, a tourist may receive an introductory certificate in as little as ten days, whereas the full program for "*Maw Nuad*" is twelve to fourteen semesters or four whole years. In the United States, we have many recognitions for Certified Thai Yoga Therapy (I.T.T.M.) Practitioners.

The Royal Thai Ministry of Health relies on the Union of Thai Traditional Medicine Society (U.T.T.S.) to formulate and maintain standards of practice and competency necessary for the formal licensing of secular, non-religious professional Traditional Thai Medicine providers in the kingdom.

Within the traditional Thai Ayurveda medical context, a Thai Yoga "*Marma Chikitsa*" therapist ("*mãw nûat*," literally, 'Traditional Marma Chikitsa Doctor') usually applies Thai Yoga together with pharmacological (herbal) or psycho-spiritual treatments as prescribed for a specific problem or specific imbalance of the Dosha or winds and humors of the body, mind, and spirit. It is becoming quite popular for many Thais to also use traditional Thai Yoga as a tool for relaxation and disease prevention rather than for a specific medical problem. However, once leaving the big city and moving into the country, there is more reliance on energy-based MedicineMedicine. This includes the resurgence and growing popularity of the self-treatment regimes and Yoga practices of "*Reusi Dotan*" or Reishi Yoga.

The term "Thai Massage" is Western slang, promoted mainly by tourists in Thailand. Although the term is now standard, it is still misunderstood and misused by the misinformed. It is easy to be confused when similar words, such as "Massage," but legally, there are distinctions and differences in definitions. Indigenous traditional Thai Yoga (I.T.T.M.), Thai Yoga Therapy, and or "Traditional Thai massage" is not the same as "Massage," "Massage Therapy," or "bodywork," as commonly defined in so-called "Massage Laws."

Please note: In standard English, when we use the word "massage," we do not mean it in the same context as the typical Western usage. In the West, "Massage" means something like a "rub down" for money and primarily refers to Swedish Massage and Massage Therapy systems. "Thai Yoga and or Thai Massage" (*Phaen Boran Ráksãa Thaang Nûat*) is entirely unrelated!

Legally words can have different meanings than words used in common, non-legal language. For example, "Massage and Massage Therapy" definitions are based on the practice of "Swedish massage." "Swedish Massage" is new (less than one hundred years) in European and American culture, and it is defined legally as "the application of a system of structured touch, pressure, movement and holding to the soft tissues of the human body to affect the health and well being of the client positively. The practice includes the external application of water, heat, cold, lubricants, salt scrubs, and other topical preparations and devices that mimic or enhance the actions of the hands."

Compare this definition with the definition given for what is Indigenous Traditional Thai Yoga (ITTM) at the beginning of this article "Thai Yoga is a comprehensive, sophisticated system of religious thera-peutics and healing arts derivative of Theraveda Buddhism, Buddhist medicine, Buddhist Psychology, Theraveda Vipassana Bhavana, Classical Indian and Tibetan Ayurveda and Yoga Vedanta. "

Indigenous Traditional Thai Yoga Therapy (Thai Massage) sounds similar to Western-style massage at first glance, but what needs to be mentioned in the proceeding definition is that Indigenous Traditional Thai yoga is a spiritually based system of healing and movement education (Yoga). It is based entirely on principles of energy balancing (Sen, Tri-Dosha, Lom, Chakra), and the actual touching, contact, or soft tissue manipulation is incidental to, and not the central aim of the practice! To emphasize this statement again, "It is possible to have a Thai Yoga session with little or no actual touching." However, touching is good! This work brings fundamental elements and energy into harmony and creates wholeness of mind, body, and spirit.

SomaVeda® Thai Yoga Therapy is a spiritually based somatic technique and profession, a modality with standards established in the Vedic and Buddhist holistic centers and temples thousands of years ago. It has an established code of ethics known as the Buddha Dharma, The Eight Fold Path, Ahimsa (non-violence), and the "Ten Rules of the Healer." There is an established criterion for education and professional practice for services, not "Massage" or "Massage therapy" as defined by secular state governments.

The SomaVeda® Thai Yoga is the core modality of our CTP(1, 2, 3), AWC, AHC, YT, TCP, Associate of Sacred Arts, and Doctorate of Sacred Natural Medicine programs. Other elements include but are not limited to Classical Indian Ayurveda, Traditional Chinese Medicine, Native American, and Western Nature Cures or Naturopathy.

NAIC Members are legally entitled to practice Native American & Thai Yoga Therapy in all fifty states without requiring special licensing. Of course, that means as long as what is practiced is not violating existing medical laws or the practice is under the umbrella of an expressive private membership associ-ation of our recognized church or ecclesiastical authority or organization. We are happy to answer any questions that are about the legal practice of our energetic and spiritually based art of healing and transformation.

Ayurvedic Thai Yoga™,
Southern Method, Supine, Session #2

Puja

Warm Up

(1) Supine Lateral Upper Leg

(2) Supine Anterior Knee

(3) Supine Lateral Lower leg

(4) Supine Anterior Foot Routine (Lang Tao)

(5) Supine Posterior Upper Leg (Ya Na Ka)

(6) Supine Medial Upper Leg (Fa Meung)

(7) Supine Medial Lower Leg

(8) Supine Inferior Foot (Fa Tao)

(9) Supine Posterior Lower Leg (Sao Nong)

(10) Supine Anterior Upper Leg
    (Raised Knee Position)

(11) Supine Anterior Lateral Upper Leg (Hurdlers Stretch)

(12) Dak Wukao (Four Positions)

(13) Supported Straight Leg

(14) Straight Leg Stretch
    (Ekapada Uttanapada Asana)

(15) Open the Wind (Bput Bpa Tu Lom)

(16) Supine Anterior Arm (Four Positions)

(17) Supine Anterior Hand (Lang Meung)

(18) Supine Posterior Hand

(1-18)---

Warm Up

Puja

Treatment Time
Work each Line 1 time: 1/2 hour
Work each Line 2 times: 1 hour
Work each Line 3 times: 1 1/2 hours

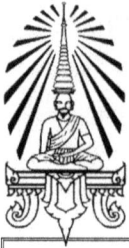

Supine Lateral Upper Leg: #1

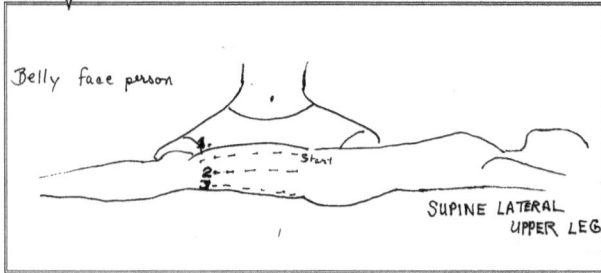

Work three lateral lines three times with rolling thumb pressure.

Indications:

Contra Indications:

Supine Anterior Knee:#2

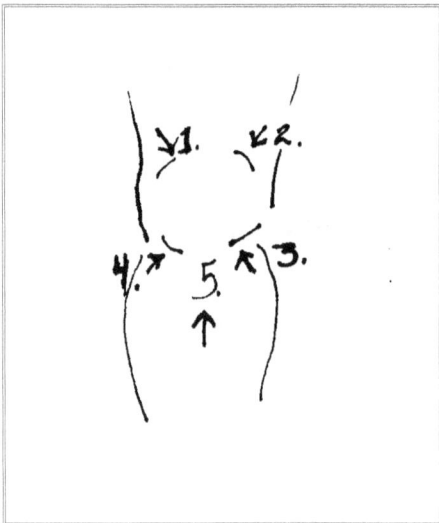

Work Five Knee Points with Reinforced Thumb Pressure.
Work in this order: Top outside, Top inside, Bottom outside, Bottom inside & Center bottom.

Indications:

Contra Indications:

Supine Lateral Lower Leg:#3

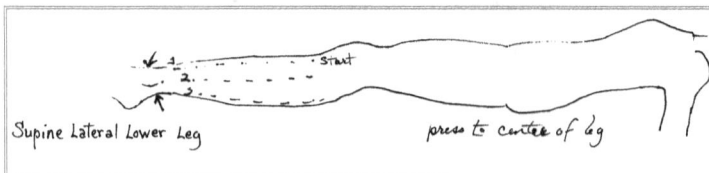

Work three lateral lines three times with rolling thumb pressure.

Indications:

Contra Indications:

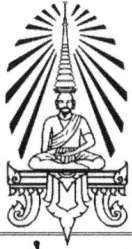

Lang Tao - Top of foot

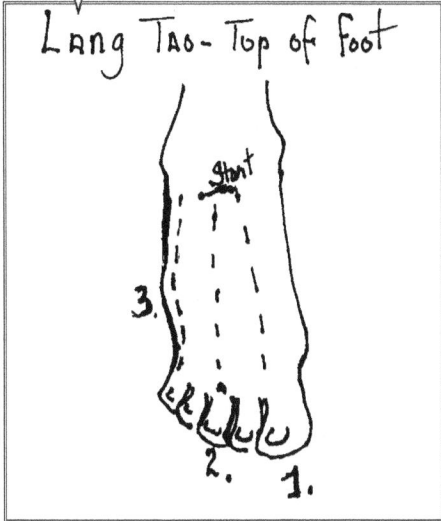

Supine Anterior Foot Routine:#4

Three Lines on top of the foot (Snake Thumb)
Circle & Pull Toes, Rotate foot/Ankle, Trist Ankle-Inward and out,
Planar flection, Dorsi flection. Remember where the toes go the
body follows.

Indications:

Contra Indications:

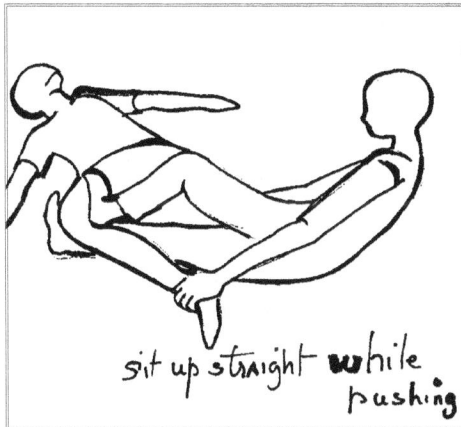

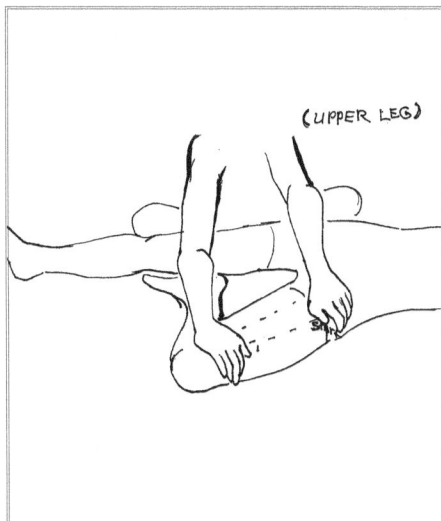

sit up straight while pushing

Supine Posterior Upper Leg:#5
(Ya Na Ka- Push the Leg)

Push the Leg in four positions with the foot.

Indications:

Contra Indications:

(UPPER LEG)

Supine Medial UpperLeg:#6

Basically "*Fa Meung*" means to Palm Press the leg. We
start here and palm press the upper inner thigh, the medial
calf and then the foot in the next two steps. Just remember,

Indications:

Contra Indications:

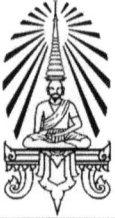

Supine Medial Lower Leg:#7

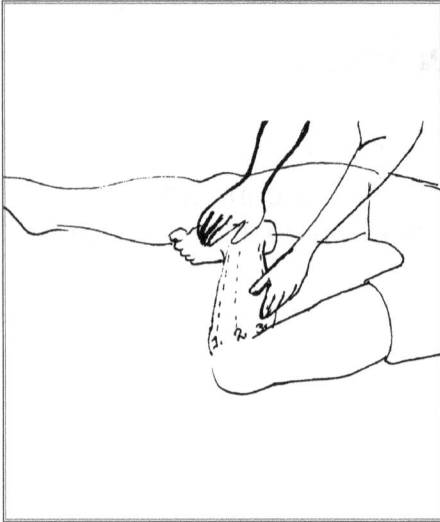

First change from your lunge into a sitting position facing the leg you are working on. Continue Fa Meung and Palm press the calf area.

_____
_____
_____

Indications:_____
Contra Indications:_____

Supine Inferior Foot:#8 (Fa Tao) Shift your position to a kneeling one beside the straight leg and facing the foot you are working on. Use thumb pressure on the two foot lines.

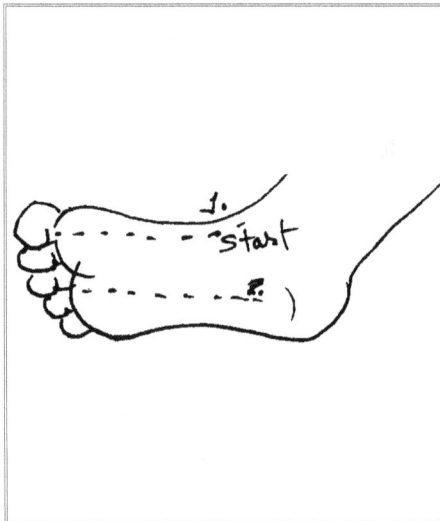

_____
_____
_____

Indications:_____
Contra Indications:_____

Supine Posterior Lower Leg:#9 (Sao Nong-Raised bent knee position)

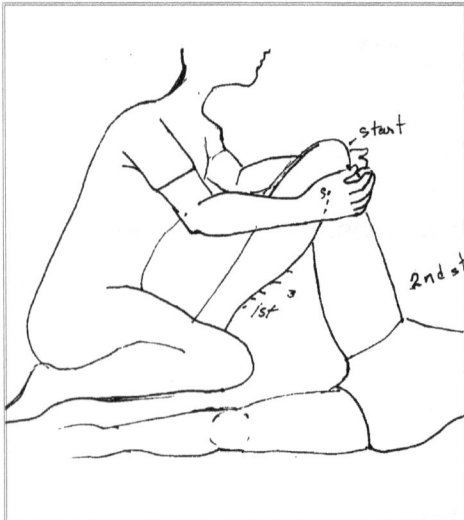

After you raise the knee, trap it securely between your knees before stretching. Hooking fingers press firmly directly behind the upper part of the lower leg.

_____
_____
_____

Indications:_____
Contra Indications:_____

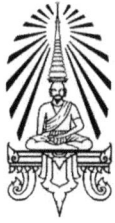

Supine Anterior Upper Leg:# 10 (Sao Nong)

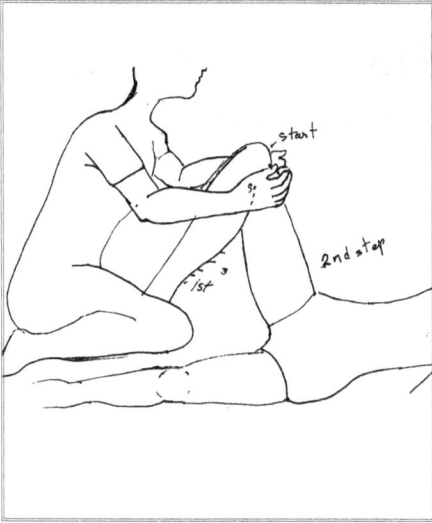

Continue with hooking fingers, walking up the front of the upper leg. Alternate pressure as you walk the line three times.

Indications:

Contra Indications:

Supine Anterior Lateral Upper Leg:#11 (Dak Kha)

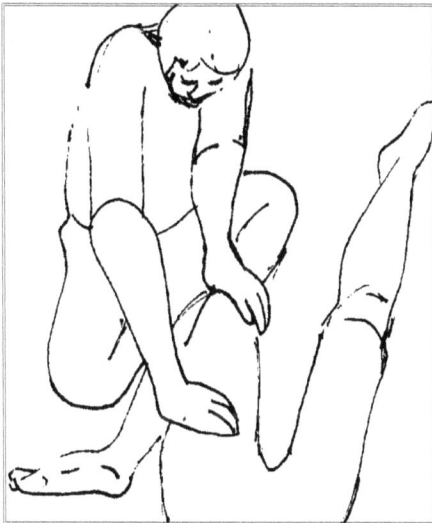

In *"Dak Kha"*, we learn to use the leverage from the whole body to lean forward and press the knee to the floor with both hands.

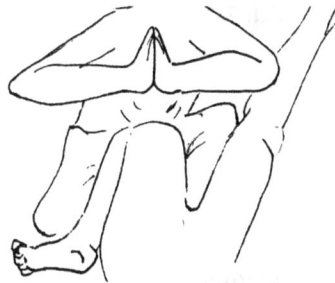

Indications:

Contra Indications:

Dak Wukao :#12 (Four Positions)

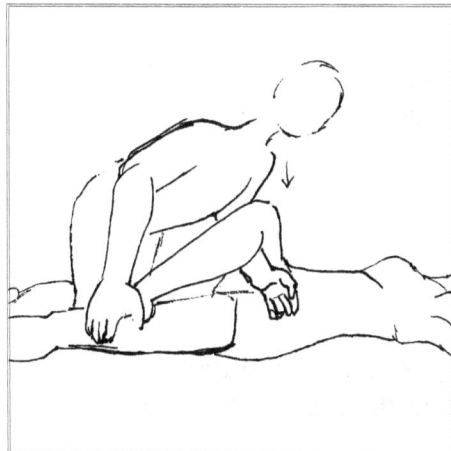

1) Upper Forearm behind knee with leverage

2) Middle Forearm behind knee with leverage

3) Wrist behind the knee with leverage

4) Come up on your knees and press with both hands.

Indications:

Contra Indications:

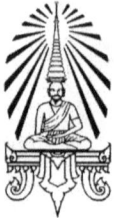

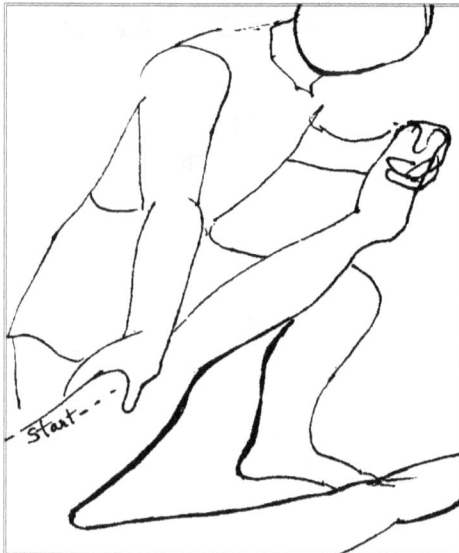

Supported Straight Leg:#13

Caution!! No direct, downward pressure on the knee
Be careful not to hyper-extend it.

_____
_____
_____
_____

Indications:_____
Contra Indications:_____

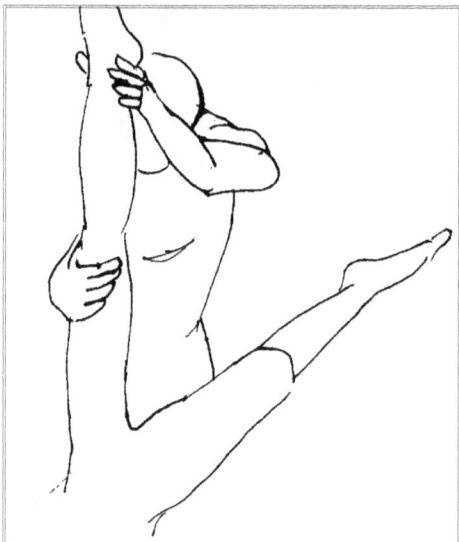

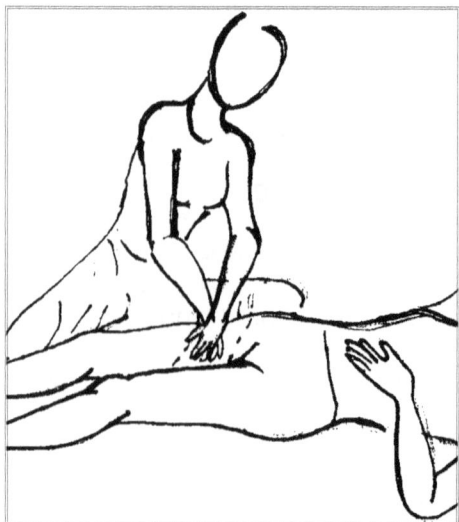

Straight Leg Stretch:#14
(Ekapada Uttanapada asana)

Keep your back and arms straight and use your body leverage
to fullest potential. Move forward if you can. Lean backwards if
the client is tight.

_____
_____
_____
_____

Indications:_____
Contra Indications:_____

Open The Wind:#15 (Bput Bpa Tu Lom)

"Open the Gate of Wind or Wind Gate". Find the Femoral
pulse, mark it and then press firmly for a ten count.
Do not move around while holding and relax.

_____
_____
_____

Indications: Diagnosed Hypertension, High Blood Pressure,
                         Blood clotting disorders. Should not be overly
Contra Indications: painful.

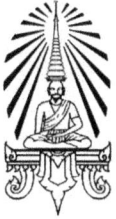

Supine Anterior Arm :#16 (Four Positions)

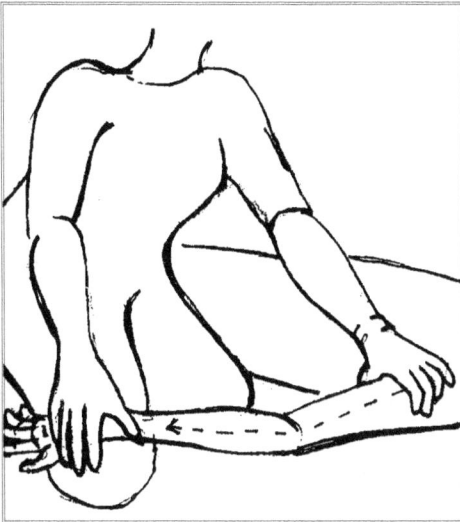

Press and hold Wind Gate "*Lom*" on top of shoulder and wrist at the same time before palm pressing entire arm as step #1.
#2. Hold Axila (Heart) point for ten count and TP medial arm.
#3Bring arm down 45degree, Alternate thumb pressure changing hands at the elbow. #4. TP Lateral arm, SIT tendons to wrist.

Indications:

Contra Indications:

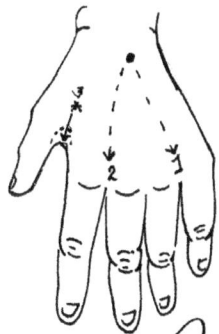

1-2. both thumbs gliding side to side (shake hand)
3. pressure from thumb and index finger for 20 seconds, release slowly toward web

Supine Anterior Hand:#17

· rub and stretch the entire palm surface between thumbs

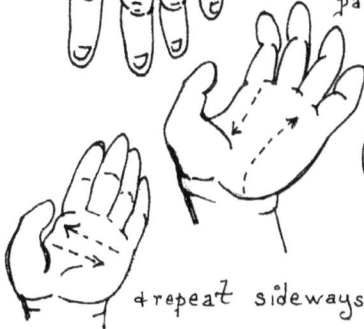

· repeat sideways

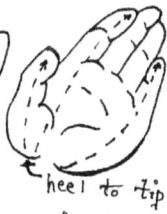

heel to tip of every finger
thumb pressure (more than one finger, if you wish ♥)

Supine Posterior Hand:#18

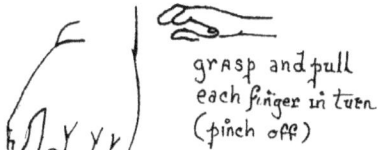

grasp and pull each finger in turn (pinch off)

dough the bread 3 times

circle and pull each finger Shake a little

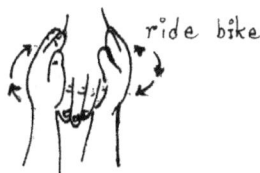

ride bike

Southern Method Side Lying Position, (S.L.P), Session #3

Puja

Warm up

(1) Side Lying Position PP, Elbow Press, TP Leg

(2) Side Lying Position Inferior Foot

(3) Side Lying Position Superior-Upper Lateral Leg

(4) Side Lying Position Hip Press and Circle

(5) Side Lying Position Lower/Middle Lamina

Groove

(6) Side Lying Position Medial Scapula

(7) Side Lying Position Upper Lamina Groove

(Lateral Cervical)

(8) Side Lying Position Lateral Cranium

(9) Side Lying Position Lateral Arm Press

(10) Side Lying Position Rotation and Stretch

(1-10)--

Warm Up

Puja

Treatment Time
Work each Line 1 time: 1/2 hour
Work each Line 2 times: 1 hour
Work each Line 3 times: 1 1/2 hours

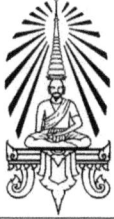

SLP Inferior Medial Leg:# 1

Lower Leg;
Palm Press
Elbow 3 pts. above the knee
Thumb Press medial line lower leg

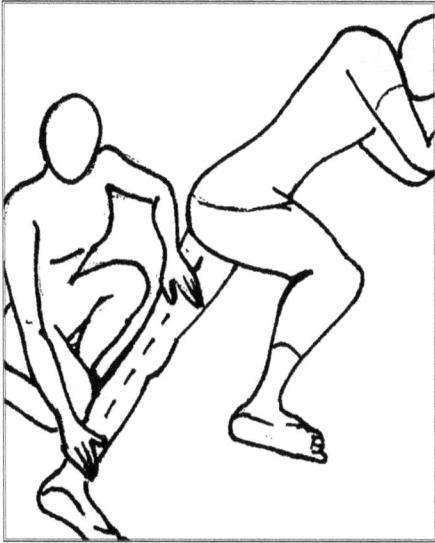

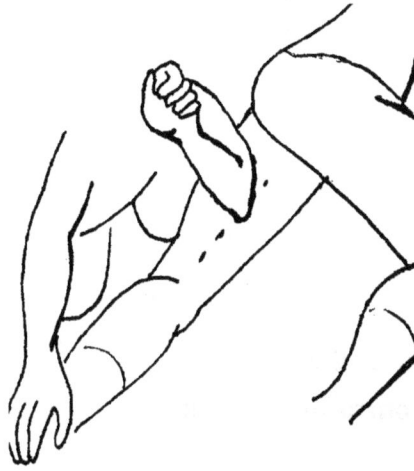

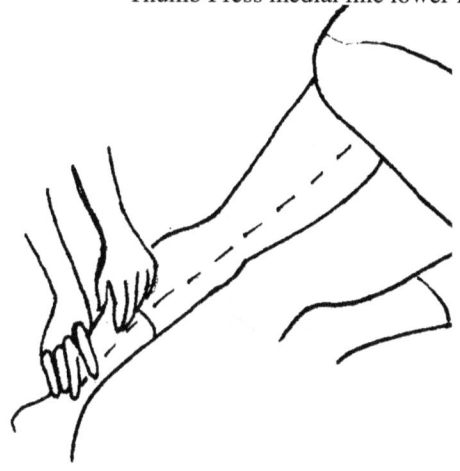

SLP Inferior Foot:#2

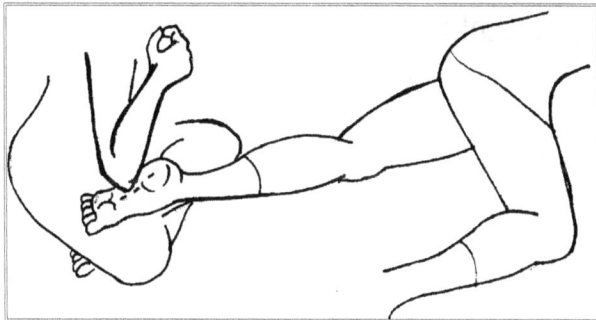

Indications: _____

Contra Indications: _____

SLP Superior Lateral Leg:#3

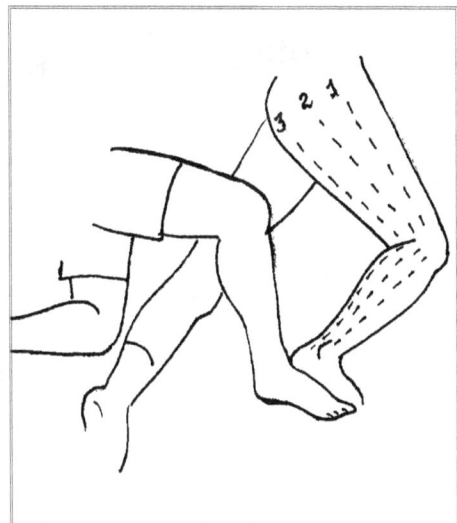

Indications: _____

Contra Indications: _____

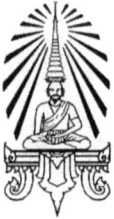

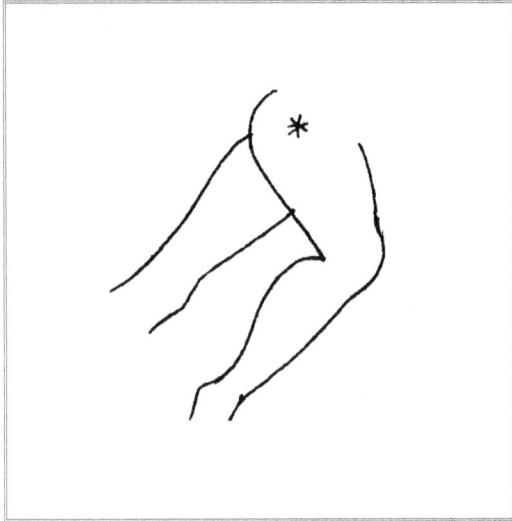

SLP Hip Palm Press & Circle:#4

_____

_____

_____

_____

Indications: _____

Contra Indications: _____

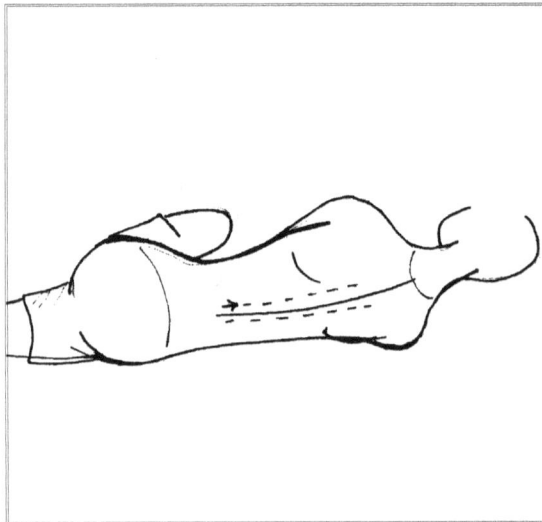

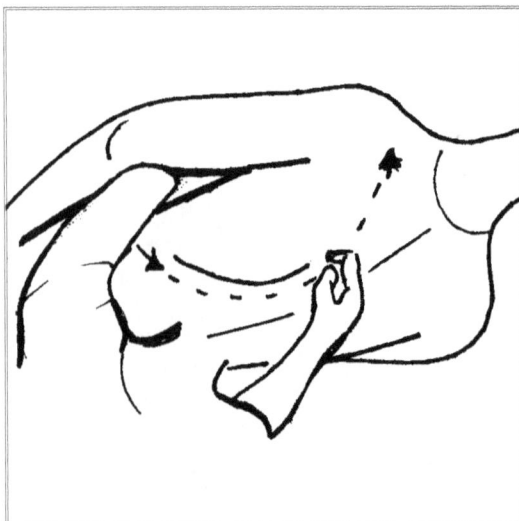

SLP Lower/Middle Lamina Groove:#5

Reinforced Rolling Thumb: 3 X

_____

_____

_____

_____

_____

_____

Indications: _____

Contra-Indications: _____

SLP Medial Scapula:#6: Broke Bird Wing

_____

_____

_____

_____

_____

_____

Indications: _____

Contra-Indications: _____

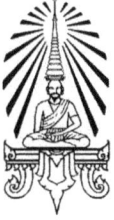

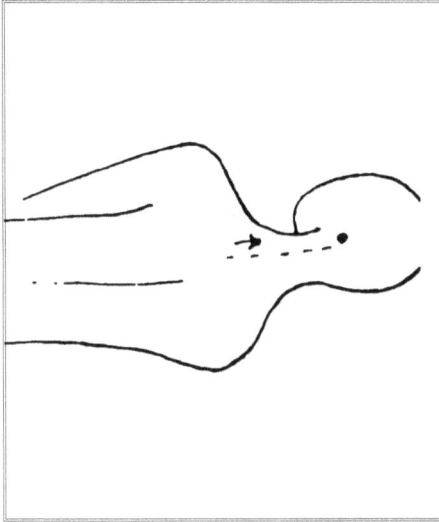

SLP Upper Lamina Groove:#7
Lunge Position Over the Head

_____
_____
_____
_____
_____

Indications: _____
Contra Indications: _____

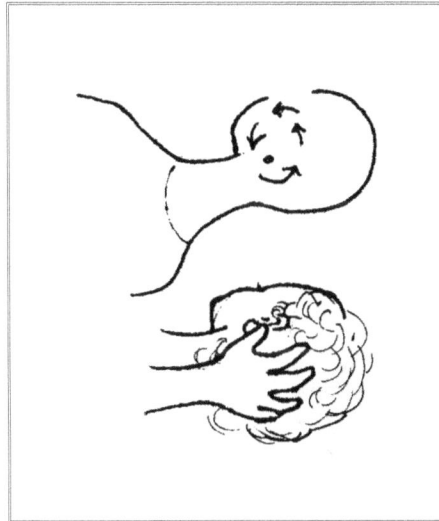

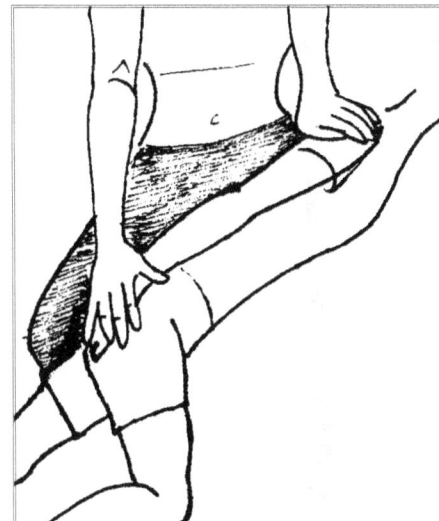

SLP Lateral Cranium:#8

Thumb Press and Thumb Circle Over and Behind the Ear

_____
_____
_____
_____
_____
_____
_____

Indications: _____
Contra Indications: _____

SLP Lateral Arm Palm Press:#9

_____
_____
_____
_____
_____
_____

Indications: _____
Contra Indications: _____

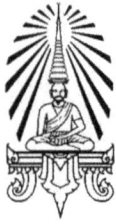

SLP Spinal Rotation & Stretch:#10

Indications: _____

Contra Indications: _____

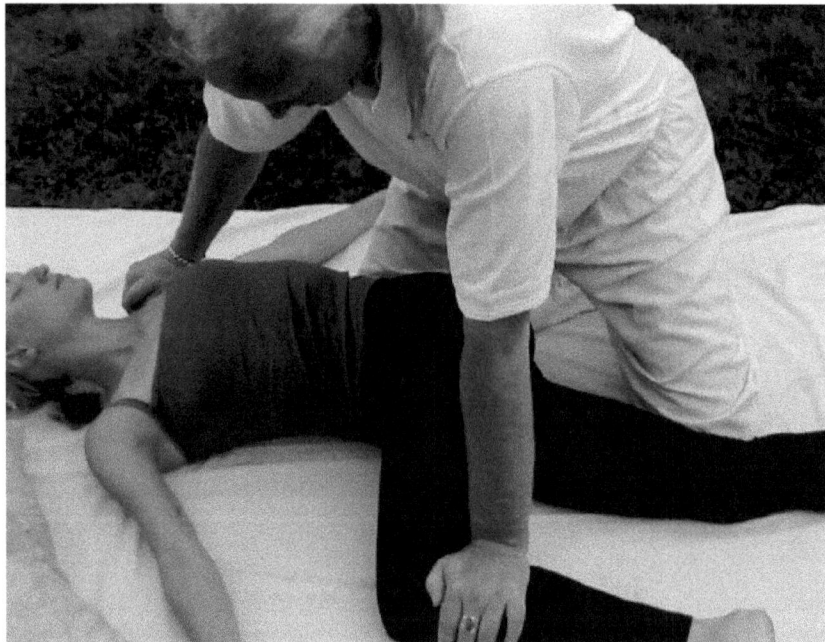

Frame Your Work Area
Keep your Head Up
Look Through Hands
Keep Your Back Straight
Keep Your Arms Straight
Rock and Breath to Create Pressure

Southern Method Prone Position, Session #4

Puja

Warm Up

    (1) Prone Torso Lamina Groove

    (2) 3 Low Back Points

    (3) Prone Lateral Scapula & Posterior Upper Arm

(2 & 3)--

    (4) Prone Posterior Leg

(4)--

    (5) Prone Torso & Gluteal Points

    (6) The Cobra Stretch (Bhujangasana)

    (6 a) Childs Pose (To release the back)

    (7) Prone Posterior Lateral Leg (Bent Knee Position)

    (8) Prone Anterior Lower Leg

(7 & 8)--

    (9) Cross Ankle & Press

(9)--

    (10) Prone Foot Press

(10)--

    (11) Toe Press (Bhekasana)

(11)--

    (12) The Half Locust (Ardis Salabhasana)

(12)--

Treatment Time
Work each Line 1 time: 1/2 hour
Work each Line 2 times: 1 hour
Work each Line 3 times: 1 1/2 hours

Warm Up

Puja

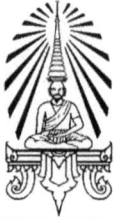

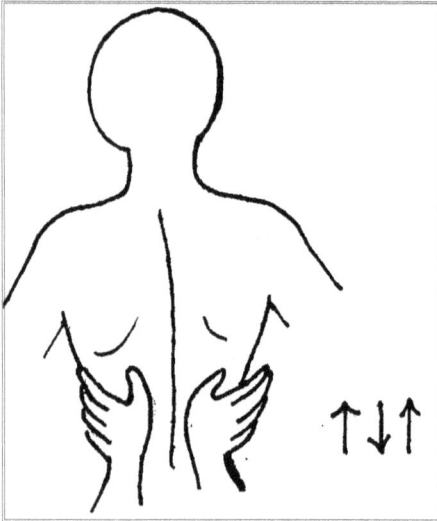

Prone Torso Lamina Groove:#1
Butterfly Palm Press

_____
_____
_____
_____

Indications:_____
Contra Indications:_____

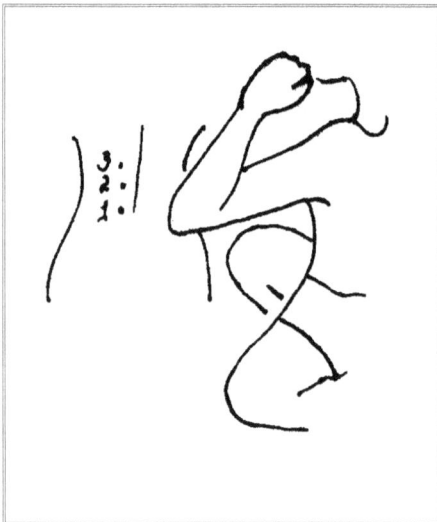

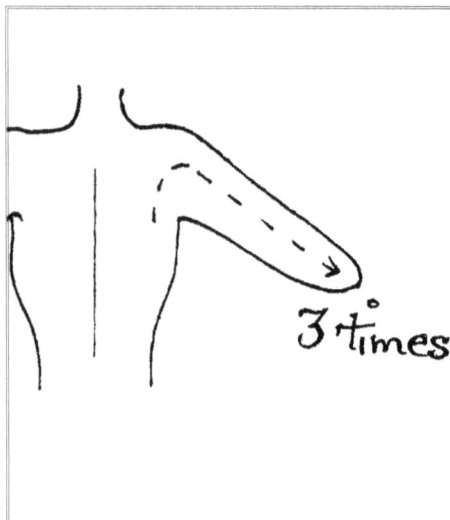

3 Low Back Points:#2
Deep Elbow Press: Caution: No pressure on the "Floating Ribs;. It is easy to crack a rib with excessive pressure here.

_____
_____
_____
_____
_____
_____

Indications:_____
Contra Indications:_____

Prone Lateral Scapula & Posterior Upper Arm: #3
Reinforced Rolling Thumb: Fold the arm upward on the side being worked to first get it out of the way and second to present to lateral Scapula and posterior arm.

_____
_____
_____
_____

Indications:_____
Contra Indications:_____

3 times

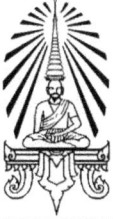

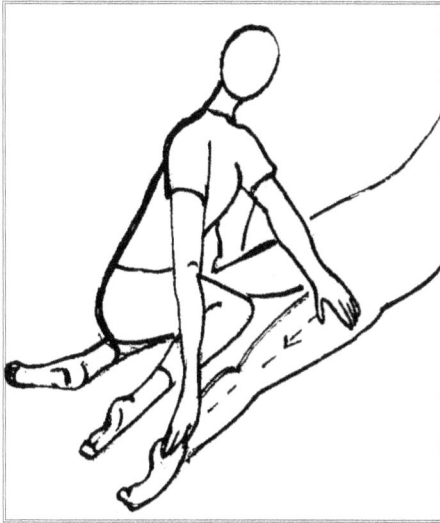

Prone Posterior Leg:#4

Palm Press Leg, Elbow Press Upper Leg Points, Thumb Press Lower Leg Points

_____

_____

_____

_____

_____

Indications: _____

Contra Indications: _____

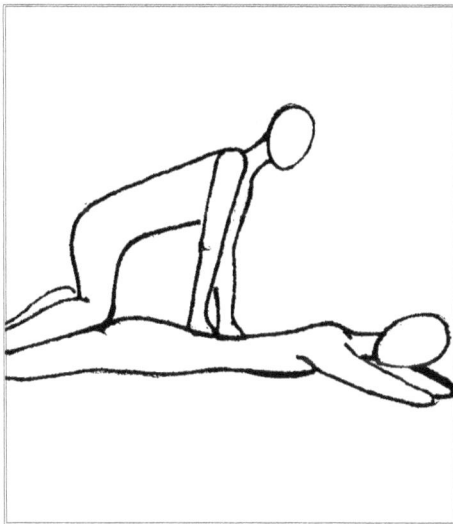

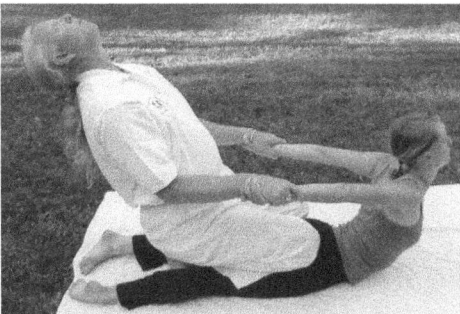

Prone Torso & Gluteal Points:#5

Position your self, kneeling on the Gluteal point , PP, PW.
Take your time and really work the back and torso well . Keep your client and yourself breathing.

_____

_____

_____

Indications: _____

Contra Indications: _____

The Cobra:#6

_____

_____

6a. Child Pose This balances and releases the Cobra. Have the client place their hands under the shoulders and press up and back onto the Knees. Guide them back into position by pulling gently on the hips. Once in position, you may do some percussion on the lower back.

Contra Indications: For Cobra use common sense, look out for rup, rods, pins, screws. Watch for integrity of the shoulders as well.

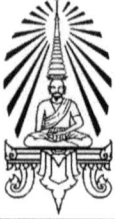

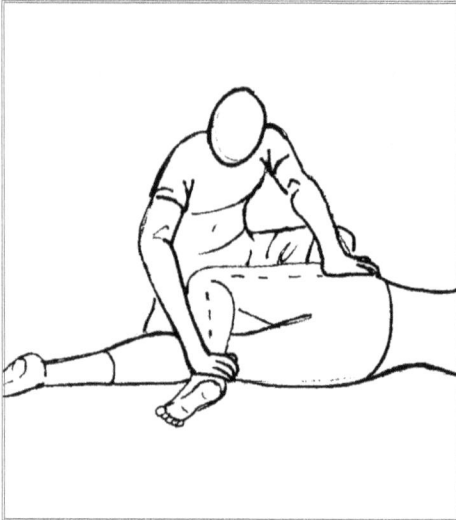

Prone Posterior Lateral Leg:#7 (Leg Stretching)

Fold the leg and place the foot of the leg being worked firmly behind the opposite knee. While pressing on the ankle work the posterior leg line from hip to ankle three times. Both hands press only one hand travels.

Indications:
Contra Indications:

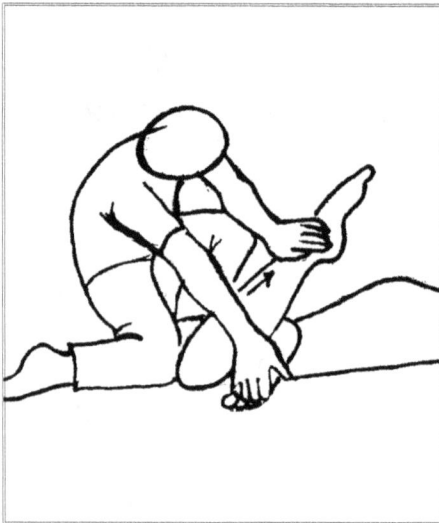

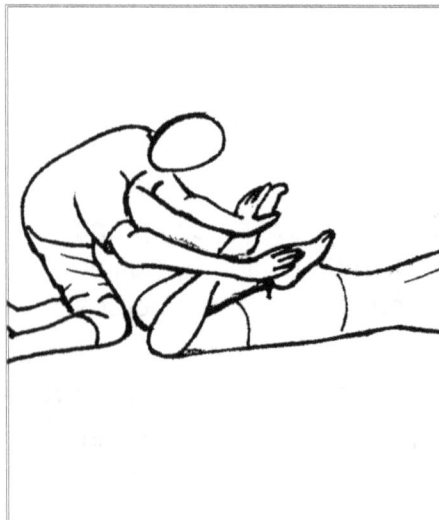

Prone Anterior Lower Leg:#8

Keeping the pressure tolerable, fold the lower leg up and over the trapped foot in the back of the knee. Palm press the three lower point on the outside (Anterior) of the lower leg. Release completly and repeat steps 7 &8 on opposite side.

Indications:
Contra Indications:

Cross Ankle & Press:#9

Indications:
Contra Indications:

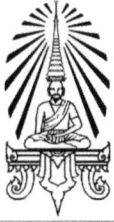

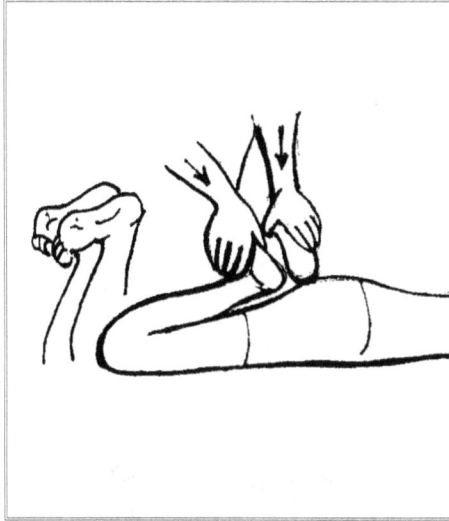

Prone Foot Press:#10

_____
_____
_____
_____
_____

Indications:_____
Contra Indications:_____

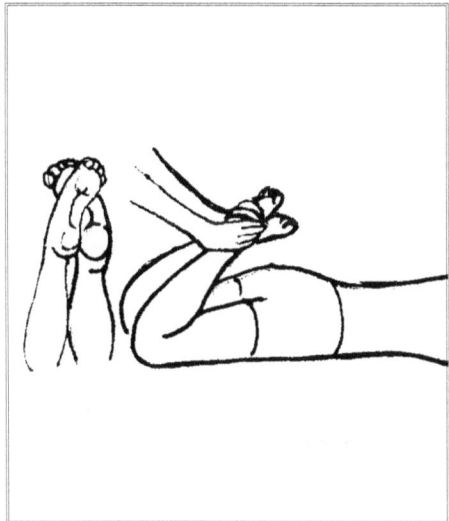

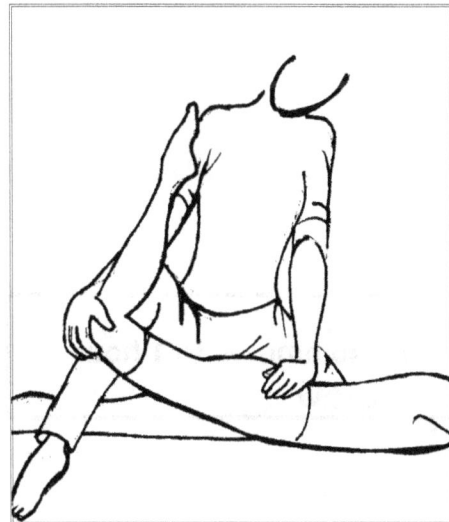

Prone Cross Toe Press:#11

_____
_____
_____
_____

Indications:_____
Contra Indications:_____

The Half Locust:#12 (Ardis Salabhasana)

Protect your back by **lifting with the legs** not your back. Work the lunge strongly, keeping your back as straight as possible. Keep your pelvis forward to lift. Feel for reasonable tension and be sensitive to client.
_____
_____
_____

Indications:_____
Contra Indications:_____

Southern Method, Second Supine Session #5
SADUNG (Stomach Focus)

Puja

Warm Up (At least 5 min.)

    (1) The Wave

    (2) Push and Pull

    (3) Five Basis Abdominal Points

    (4) Abdominal Press

    (5) Anterior Torso

    (6) Supine Medial Upper Leg (Figure Four over Knee)

    (7) Supine Cross Leg Spinal Rotation

(6 & 7)---

    (8) Supine Posterior Upper Leg and Crossed Leg
      Combined

 (8)--

    (9) Supine Inferior Foot (Standing Position)

 (9)--

    (10) Supported Shoulder Stand

    (11) Straight Leg Pull-up

    (12) The Plow(Halasana)

    (13) Cross Leg Pull-up

Warm Up

Puja

Treatment time: 45minutes to 1 hour
Slow

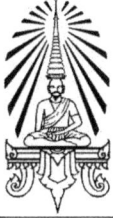

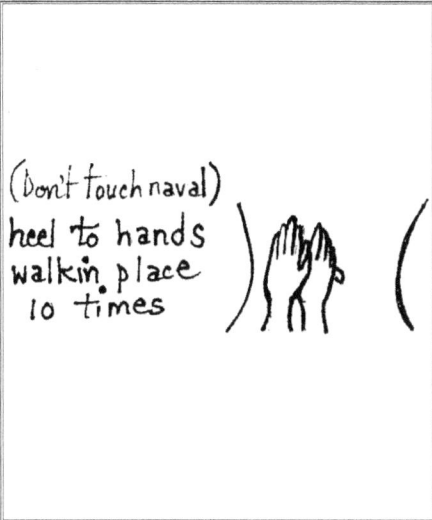

(Don't touch naval)
heel to hands
walkin place
10 times

The Wave:#1

Before Wave technique. arm up the abdoman by gentle 30 to 108 Palm circles around the Hara. Do Wave 10 times clockwise.

Indications:

Contra Indications: Appendicitus, extreme Collitus, ruptured Colon, Abdominal Cancer, Abdominal infections

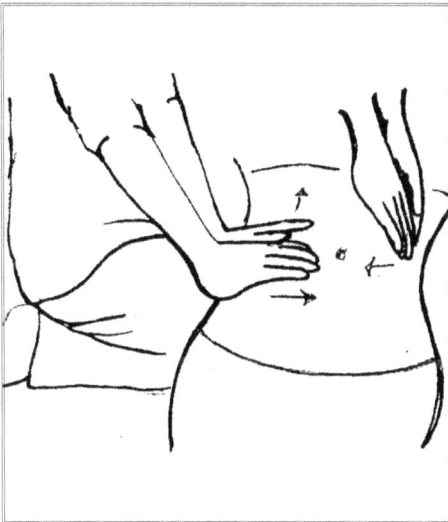

Push and Pull:#2

Push and pull, rocking from the heel of the palms over to the finger tips. Imagine the center lline on the abdomen and skip over it - not touching. The angle for the pressure should be about 45 degree down and inward toward the spine.

Indications:

Contra Indications:

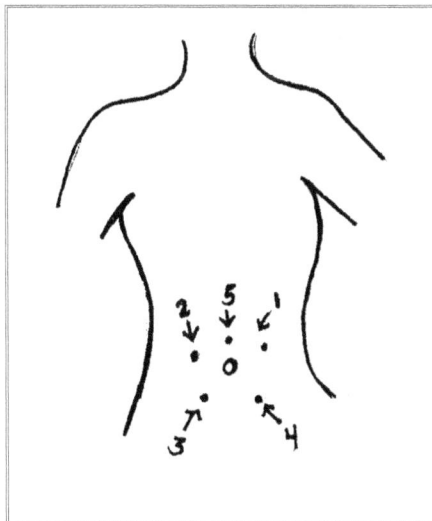

Five Basic Abdominal Points:#3

Indications:

Contra Indications:

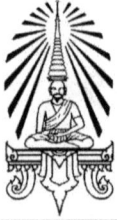

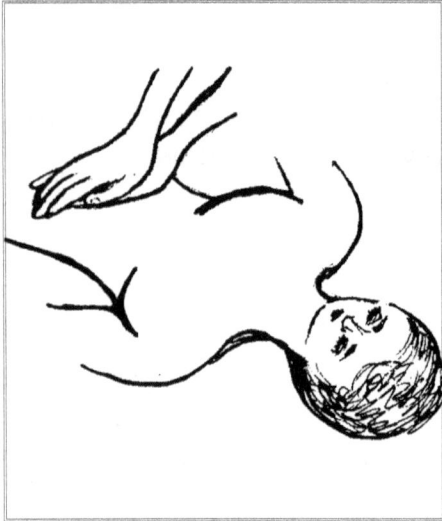

Abdominal Press:#4

Indications:
Contra Indications:

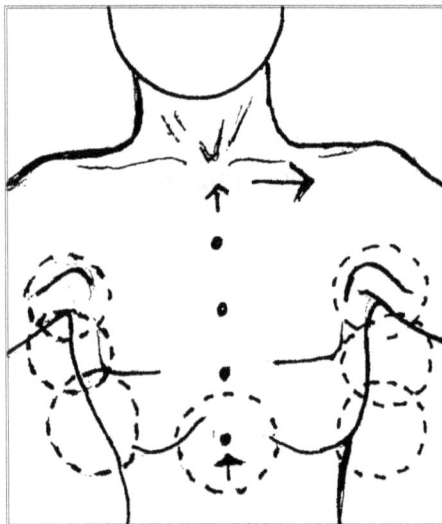

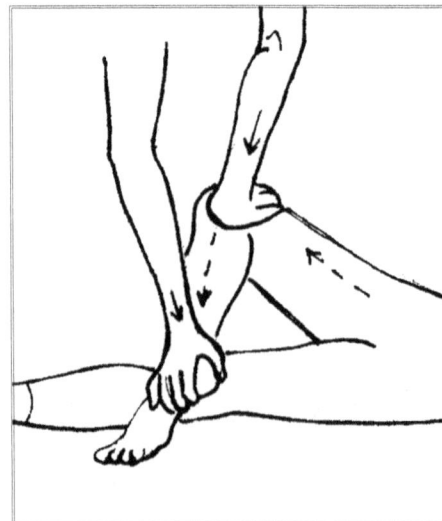

Anterior Torso:#5

Use finger tip pressure to make generous figure eight circles up the sternum and around the chest.

Indications:
Contra Indications:

Supine Medial Upper Leg: #6

Figure Four Over Knee: Toe and Knee Press

Indications:
Contra Indications:

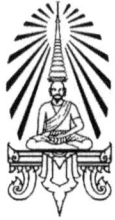

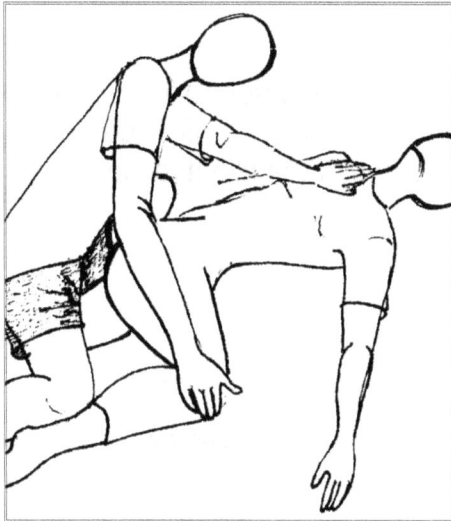

Supine Cross Leg Spinal Rotation:#7

Indications:

Contra Indications:

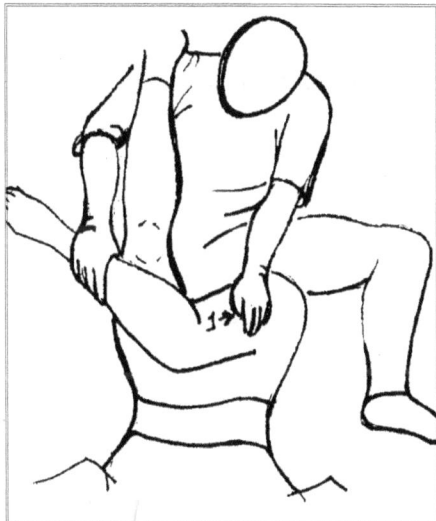

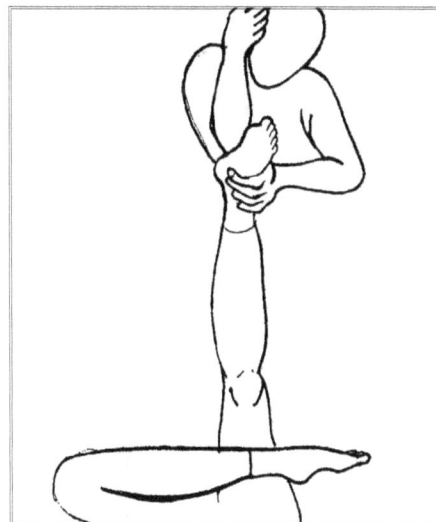

Supine Posterior UpperLeg and Crossed Leg Combined:#8

Indications:

Contra Indications:

Supine Inferior foot (Standing Position):#9

A) Lever the leg strongly. Doing a good range of motion here makes the next part easier and less painful.
B) Elbow press the bottom of the foot while locking the toes downward firmly.

Indications:

Contra Indications:

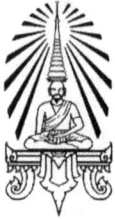

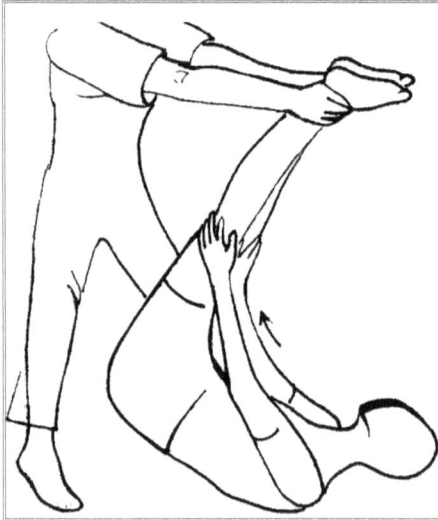

Supported Shoulder Stand:#10

Use a strong three part lift: 1) Pull to your abdomen 2) Turn and look 3) Push into balance position. With practice do all three motions in one smooth lift. Keep the arms of the client locked and make sure they are breathing.

Indications:

Contra Indications: Pay attention to neck and upper back problems.

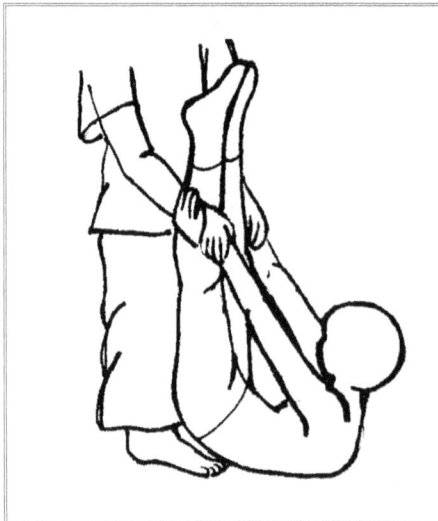

Straight Leg Pull Up:#11

Bend your knees and lift with the legs. Do this pull up with only back strength and you will be the next client!

Indications:

Contra Indications:

The Plow (Halasana):#12

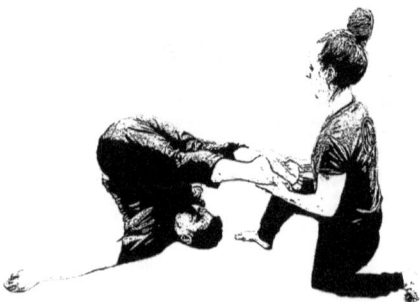

Indications:

Contra Indications:

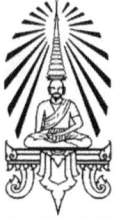

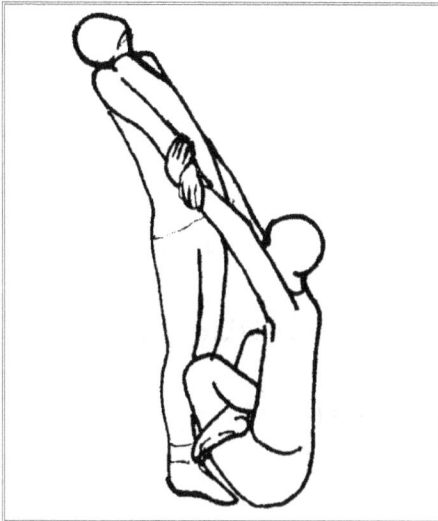

Crossed Leg Pull Up:#13

_____

_____

_____

_____

Indications: _____

Contra Indications: _____

Body Mechanics and Angle of Attack:

The higher the point or line being worked relative to the specific body part and the floor, the higher the center of gravity relative to it. The lower or more Acute the point is relative to the body part and floor, the lower the working center of gravity.

Stated; If the lines are on top, so are you! If the line is on the side, go low!

THERE ARE NO MISTAKES IN SomaVeda® ONLY POSSIBILITIES For FURTHER REFINEMENTS!

Southern Method, Seated Position, Session #6

Puja

Warm Up

(1) Seated Position Posterior Upper Torso

(a) Thumb press between Shoulders (up, down, up)

(b) Thumb press along top of Shoulders (out, back, out)

(c) Thumb press Posterior Cervical (unilateral, 3X)

(d) Cranial Lift (Cranial base points: Bilateral))

(e) Finger circle Temples (both sides- Bilateral)

(f) Thumb press Governing Vessal (Klai Sen- Snake)

(2) Seated Position Neck Rotation (Namaskar Mudra)

(3) Seated Position Seventh Chakra Release (Standing)

(4) Seated Position Reinforced Upper Torso Rotation

(5) Seated Position Spinal Push (BiLateral Knee)(1,2,1)

(6) Seated Position Full Forward Bend

(Paschimottanasana) (Lunge position: Palm Press: 1, 2, 3, 2, 1- Unilateral)

(7) Seated Position Facial Treatment (12 Lines)

Warm Up

Puja

Treatment Time
Rapid - 20 minutes
Slow - 45 min..

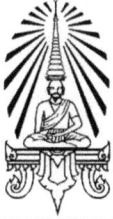

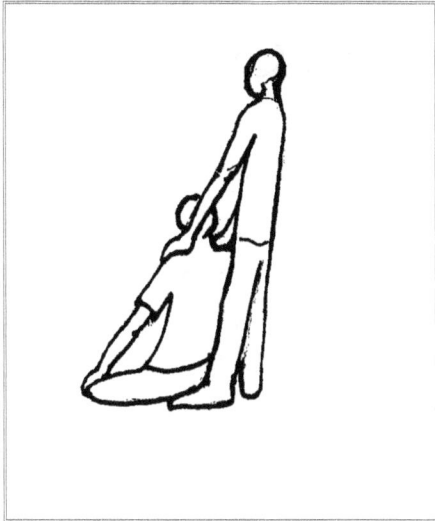

Seated Position Posterior Torso:#1

Warm up the shoulders with some Palm Pressing along the top.
a) TP between the shoulders
b) TP on top of shoulders
c) TP posterior cervical
d) Cranial Lift
e) Finger circles on temples
f)TP Governing Vessal

Indications:

Contra Indications:

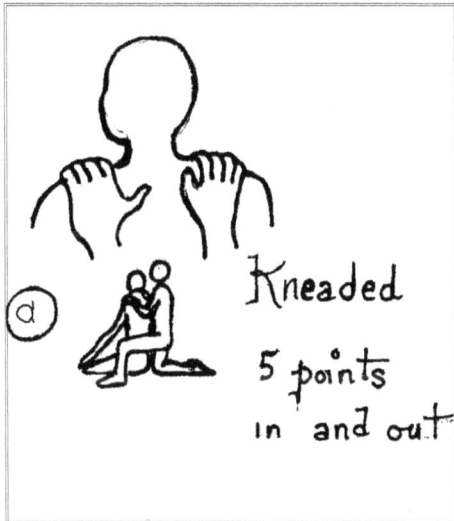

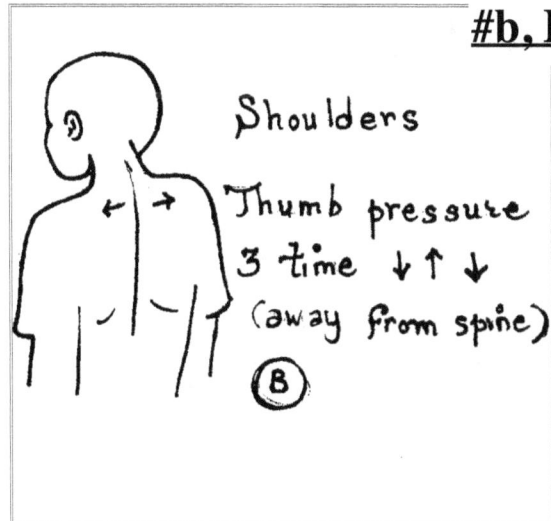

#a, Thumb Press along top of Shoulders

Kneaded

5 points
in and out

Indications:

Contra Indications:

#b, PP & Thumb Press between Shoulders:

Shoulders

Thumb pressure
3 time ↓↑↓
(away from spine)
Ⓑ

Indications:

Contra Indications:

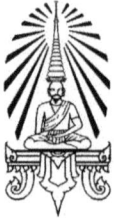

Rolling Thumb Pressure
3 times ↑ ↓ ↑

7 points
press away from s[pine]

Change sides and
work opposite side
equally.

Thumb Press Posterior Cervical:#c

Indications:_____

Contra Indications:_____

Cranial Lift

Raise head upright
with thumbs on the
cranial base points.
fingers on temporal area,
lift cranium 5 seconds
and release slowly.

Cranial Lift:#d

Indications:_____

Contra Indications:_____

Finger Circle Temples:#e

Massage
circular
digital
pressure

Indications:_____

Contra Indications:_____

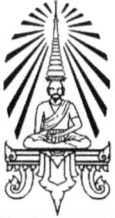

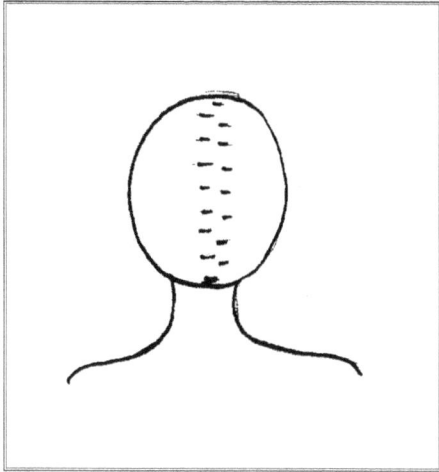

Thumb Press Governing Vessal (KlaiSen):

_____
_____
_____
_____
_____
_____

Indications: _____
Contra Indications: _____

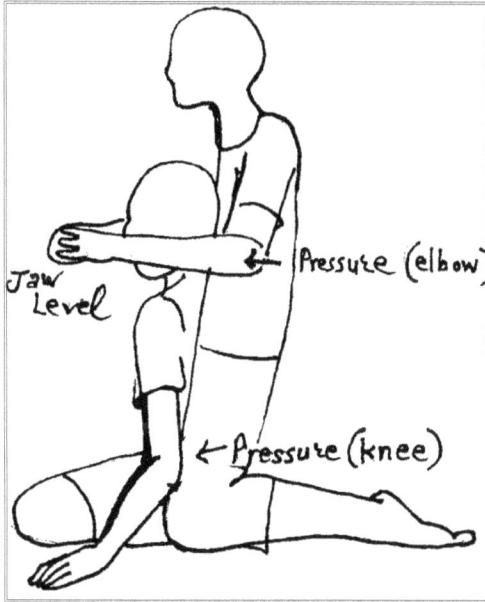

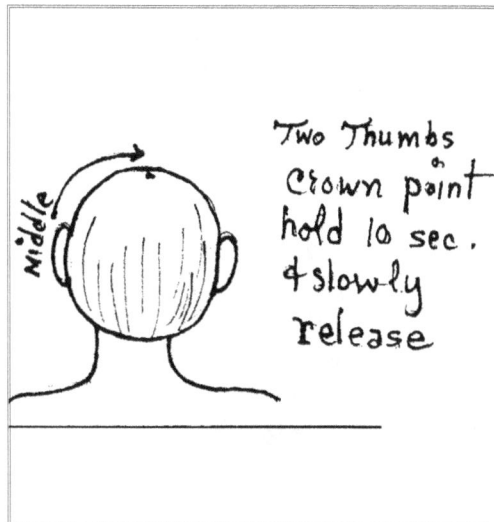

Seated Position Neck Rotation:#2

Jaw Level
Pressure (elbow)
Pressure (knee)

_____
_____
_____
_____

Indications: _____
Contra Indications: _____

Seated Position Seventh Chakra Release: #3

Middle

Two Thumbs
on Crown point
hold 10 sec.
& slowly
release

_____
_____
_____

Indications: _____
Contra Indications: _____

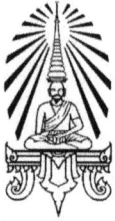

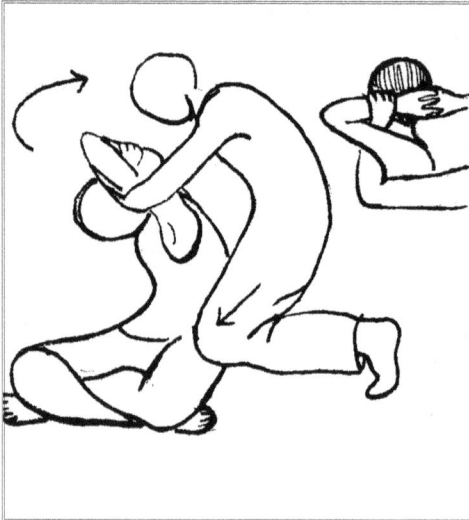

Reinforced Upper Torso Rotation:#4

_____
_____
_____
_____
_____

Indications: _____
ContraIndications: _____

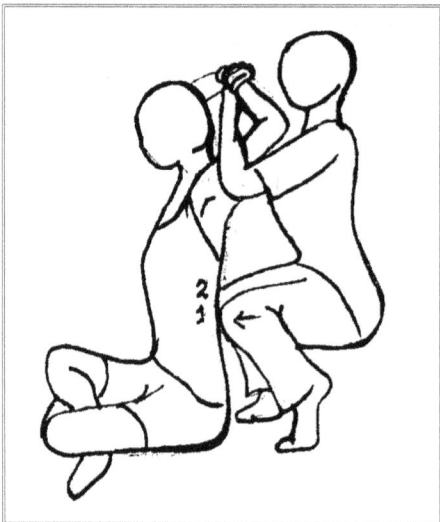

Spinal Push (BiLateralKnee):#5

_____
_____
_____
_____
_____

Indications: _____
ContraIndications: _____

FullForwardBend:#6 (Paschimottanasana)

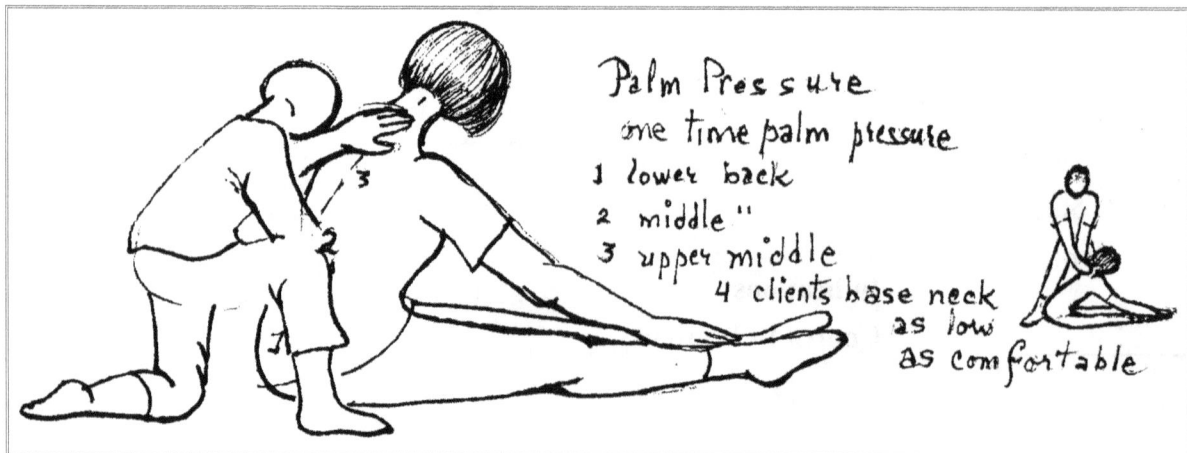

Palm Pressure
one time palm pressure
1 lower back
2 middle "
3 upper middle
    4 clients base neck
    as low
    as comfortable

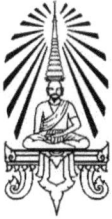

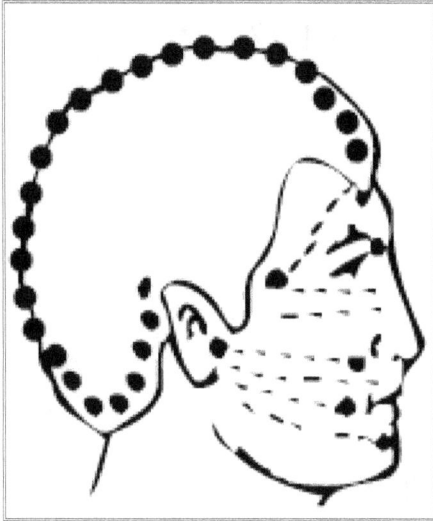

Facial Treatment:#7

_____
_____
_____
_____
_____
_____
_____

Indications: _____

Contraindications: _____

Relax
Frame Your Work Area
Keep your Head Up
Look Through Arms-Hands
Keep Your Back Straight
Keep Your Arms Straight
Rock and Breathe to Create Pressure

The SomaVeda®
Therapeutic day

Southern Method, General Session #1 and #7

Puja

(A) Supine Position

    (1) Supine Lateral Upper Leg

    (2) Supine Anterior Knee

    (3) Supine Lateral Lower leg

    (4) Supine Anterior Foot Routine (Lang Tao)

    (5) Supine Posterior Upper Leg (Ya Na Ka)

    (6) Supine Medial Upper Leg (Fa Meung)

    (7) Supine Medial Lower Leg

    (8) Supine Inferior Foot (Fa Tao)

    (9) Supine Posterior Lower Leg (Sao Nong)

    (10) Supine Anterior Upper Leg

       (Raised Knee Position)

    (11) Supine Anterior Lateral Upper Leg

    (12) Dak Wukao (Four Positions)

    (13) Supported Straight Leg

    (14) Straight Leg Stretch

      (Ekapada Uttanapada Asana)

    (15) Open the Wind (Bput Bpa Tu Lom)

    (16) Supine Anterior Arm (Four Positions)

    (17) Supine Anterior Hand (Lang Myung)

    (18) Supine   Posterior Hand

(1-18)--

(B) Side Lying Position

(1) Side Lying Position Inferior Medial Upper Leg

(2) Side Lying Position Inferior Foot

(3) Side Lying Position Superior Lateral Leg

(4) Side Lying Position Hip Press and Circle

(5) Side Lying Position Lower/Middle Lamina Groove

(6) Side Lying Position Medial Scapula

(7) Side Lying Position Upper Lamina Groove

(Lateral Cervical)

(8) Side Lying Position Lateral Cranium

(9) Side Lying Position Lateral Arm Press

(10) Side Lying Position Rotation and Stretch

(1-10)--

Work each Line 1 time: 1/2 hour
Work each Line 2 times: 1 hour
Work each Line 3 times: 1 1/2 hour

(C) Prone Position

(1) Prone Torso Lamina Groove

(2) 3 Low Back Points

(3) Prone Lateral Scapula & Posterior Upper Arm

(2 & 3)--

(4) Prone Posterior Leg

(4)--

(5) Prone Torso & Gluteal Points

(6) The Cobra Stretch (Bhujangasana), (6a) Child Pose

(7) Prone Posterior Lateral Leg (Bent Knee Position)

(8) Prone Anterior Lower Leg

(7 & 8)---

(9) Cross Ankle & Press

(9)---

(10) Prone Foot Press

(10)---

(11) Toe Press (Bhekasana)

(11)---

(12) The Half Locust (Artis Salabhasana)

(12)---

(D) Second Supine Position

1) The Wave

(2) Push and Pull

(3) Five Basis Abdominal Points

(4) Abdominal Press

(5) Anterior Torso

(6) Supine Medial Upper Leg (Crossed Position)
(7) Supine Cross Leg Stretch

(6 & 7)---

(8) Supine Posterior Upper Leg and Crossed Leg
    Combined

(8)---

(9) Supine Inferior Foot (Standing Position)

(9)---

    (10) Supported Shoulder Stand

    (11) Straight Leg Pull-up

    (12) The Plow (Halasana)

    (13) Cross Leg Pull-up

(E) Seated Position

    (1) Seated Position Posterior Upper Torso

        (a) Thumb press between Shoulders

        (b) Thumb press along top of Shoulders

        (c) Thumb press Posterior Cervical

        (d) Cranial Lift

        (e) Finger circle temples

        (f) Thumb press Governing Vessel (Klai Sen)

    (2) Neck Rotation

    (3) Seventh Chakra Release

    (4) Reinforced Upper Torso Rotation

    (5) Spinal Push (BiLateral Knee)

    (6) Full Forward Bend (Paschimottanasana)

    (7) Facial Treatment

Puja

Treatment Time
Work each Line 1 time: 1 hour
Work each Line 2 times: 1 1/2 hours
Work each Line 3 times: 2 + hours

SomaVeda Integrated Traditional Therapies®

We offer training from beginner to Master!

Current NAIC program offerings in the US:
1) Certified SomaVeda® Thai Yoga Practitioner: CTP1 (A 164 CE hour residential training)
2) Certified Ayurveda Wellness Counselor: CTP2 (A 200 CE hour residential training)
3) Certified Ayurveda Health Consultant: CTP3 (A 200 CE hour residential training)
4) Certified SomaVeda® Thai Yoga Teacher: TCP1 (An 1008 CE hour residential training)
5) Doctor of Sacred Natural Medicine Program (DSNM/ ND)(Naturopathic Board Eligibility Course)
    (A 2595 hour certification program qualifying graduates to sit for the ANCB Naturopathic National Boards. Includes both in class residential programs and distance learning modules)
6) Doctor of Sacred Traditional and Indigenous Medicine (D.S.T.I.M.) Fast Track "*BareBones*" Degree in eigth to twelve months!

For details on any of the above program and certification courses ask your instructor or visit our school website at https://www.SomaVeda.Org.

SomaVeda® Continuing Education and Practice Building Courses:

1) https://LearnThaiYoga.Teachable.com

Current International Training, Tour and Certification Courses:

1) https://ThailandStudyTours.Com
    (Thai Ministry approved certifications.)

Thai Yoga, Thai Massage Books, DVD, Home Study Courses, Genuine Thai Yoga Mats:

1) https://BeardedMedia.Com

SomaVeda® Thai Yoga and Thai Massage Products: T-Shirts, Clothing, Posters, Gifts etc.
Official Logo Thai Yoga Center School Uniforms:
1) https://BeardedMedia.Com

Let's connect:
INSTAGRAM: @thaiyogacenter
https://www.instagram.com/thaiyogacenter/

FACEBOOK: https://www.facebook.com/anthony.james.733076/
Thai Yoga Center: https://thaiyogacenter.com
SomaVeda College of Natural Medicine: https://somaveda.org
Learn Thai Yoga Online! https://learnthaiyoga.teachable.com
Native American Indigenous Church Tribal Organization: https://somaveda.com

Visit Exotic THAILAND
December 7th. to December 19th. 2023!

Early register and save! Sign up now and Receive over $5,295.00 in FREE Bonus Materials!!

Sacred Sites & Mystical Places

We are excited about our expanded schedule and services.

This year we have expanded our schedule to include at least four different opportunities to experience Thailand with our small group format. As usual ,we will be basing our program on a Cultural Immersion/ Eco-Tour type of approach. We spend a significant portion of our program time working with indigenous teachers and professional Thais, in actually experiencing and learning traditional Thai healing arts and culture. We have the experience and commitment to having your experience in the kingdom of Thailand to be the very best. This is the very same program to be awarded the "Friend of Thailand Award" from the national gov't of Thailand. This is the only western based program to be so honored and now you can be a part of it!

Thailand is described by most travelers as the most exotic country on the planet. Nowhere else succeeds quite so well blending an age old culture of rich heritage and traditions, with the developments and advantages of the modern world. Tradition and cultural heritage is at the very core ' daily life for the Thai people. Totally at peace with themselves and their world, there is a cheerfulness that is forever present in the faces of nearly everyone you meet.

NAIC, Inc.., Ajahn, Anthony B. James Traditional Thai Healing Art & Sacred Sites Practicum/ Tour In Thailand, December 7th. to December 19th. 2023 , Two weeks in Thailand! Uthai Thani, Bangkok, Ayudthaya.

This is the only NAIC recommended and Approved Thailand Program awarding recognized CEU's. (NTYMBCB Cat. A)

You are invited to experience firsthand "The Practical Expression of Loving Kindness" in the land of its origin. Over the next thirteen (13) days we will explore the profound spiritual roots of SomaVeda® Traditional Thai Yoga in the actual temples and schools credited with preserving its heritage. This is not just a guided tour. Dr. Anthony B. James will be facilitating a comprehensive training and immersion experience. Participants gain a minimum of 100 hrs. to of course credit (CEU's) in SomaVeda®, (Buddhai Sawan/ SriPai). Thailand certification program. The program is a total survey of traditional and modern practice and applications including institutional as well as traditional massage of Thailands native peoples and authentic Monastic traditional medicine. There will be a special training session in Royal Thai approved program under patronage and recognition of the Thai Monks! NAIC is the only western based program with permission to do this training! We will also be doing internship with a famous hospital under the supervision of one of Thailands most famous doctors!

There is no prerequisite for participation. We will study, train, practice, walk, explore, receive hands on traditional sessions in a variety of styles, meditate, visit vortices of healing energy thousands of years old, we will eat well, study more, practice more, laugh, cry and prosper in love, compassion, joy and equanimity. To prepare you for your journey Dr. James has prepared a comprehensive packet including what to bring, what to wear, food tips and source materials on Thailand's religion, art and culture. Now is your opportunity to become part of the international community of SomaVeda® Therapist.

There is no better way to immerse yourself into SomaVeda® Thai Massage than to experience a total immersion training tour in Thailand!!

Want to take some beautiful pictures? EXPECT TO SEE: Uthai Thani District and town, Bangkok or Krungthep, Grand Palace, Wat Phra Kaew - Temple of the Emerald Buddha and Royal Chapel, the spectacular Royal Collection of Weapons and the Coin pavilion. The Amulet Market, Wat Po, (the popular name for Wat Pra Chetupon), the original home for our school Wat Buddhai Sawan in Ayudthaya, We have arranged for lessons in hands on healing and Traditional Thai "Tok Sen" Nuad with elders in the village as well. We have special arrangements to be some of the very first western students to train with a famous blind Master healer!

ThailandStudyTours.Com to Register!

There is no better way than this to bring authenticity to your oriental and Thai style practice. Immerse yourself in Thai culture. Study Traditional Thai Medical Massage with Grand Master's and teacher's as well as Master Instructor Ajahn, Dr. Anthony B. James. Why consider going to Thailand without instructors who speak Thai and English? For the cultural and artistic minded , participants receive additional intensive instruction in the classic and folk art styles unique to Thailand from North to South.

Interested in Sacred Relics? It's one thing to read about these sacred places ... it's quite another to visit them first hand with a master to guide you!

This Fantastic Thirteen (13) day excursion is valued at $4,595.00. However, sign up by June 11th., 2023 for only $3,385.00. In fact everything you need is included except International Airfare/ Transpotation, food and personal shopping.

Additionally including over $5,200.00 in Free Bonus Materials!! (Details on website at https://ThailandStudyTours.Com)

* The trip is currently limited with several slots already committed. . Pay full price after August 8th, 2023, unless Early Bird registration is extended. All prices subject to change at any time without notice. No price guarantee of any kind without a deposit. The minimum deposit $600.00 USD. Deposits and payments may now be made in real time through our secure Paypal or Google Checkout accounts.

YES, I WANT TO GO! I realize seating is limited and request to reserve a place on this fantastic adventure. What could be better, fun and course credit!

Yes, I want to pay a deposit, save an extra $5,200.00 in discounts and bonuses and to secure my seat for this incredible trip! .

Reserve your seat today! (706) 358-8646
E-Mail nativeaic@somaveda.com
WebSite: https://ThailandStudyTours.Com

** **See the complete itinerary and Waiver/ Agreement** for exhaustive details. Price is set with deposit, otherwise is subject to change at any time. Please Note: Although this trip is designed for students, it is well supervised and chaperoned by our staff. Classes are not taught by just anyone--they are all taught by Certified and recognized Master Instructors. All of our guides are   professionally licensed and insured by the Thai Government. Most if not all are Thai Citizens with college degrees in related Humanities. This is NOT a classic budget trip/carry your own food sleep where you can/ get by as best you can (maybe) type of excursion- which some other less experienced agents may be offering. Do not settle for less than the best! If they are offering free accommodations or travel, you can bet there is some corner cutting somewhere!

If your considering another excursion ask them do they provide bonded, licensed drivers, do they provide their own vehicles? Do they expect you to share bathing and shower accommodations? Do they guarantee exactly who all their staff are, and their level of professional certification? Are they insured? Will an owner of the company be accompanying the group and will there always be someone available to translate Thai and English as necessary?

We do cover all of these issues and more. With over thirtynine years experience in Thailand and the local first class resources that we have developed we can guarantee a great experience. And a SAFE ONE!